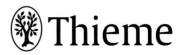

Tuina Therapy

Treatment of Adults and Children

Weizhong Sun, MD
Chief Consultant
Medical Director
German Tuina Academy
Bad Füssing, Germany
Guest Professor
University for TCM
Shandong, China

Arne Kapner, MD†
Former Head of Therapy Center
German Center for Osteoporosis
Johannesbad Clinic
Bad Füssing, Germany

261 illustrations

Thieme
Stuttgart · New York

Library of Congress Cataloging-in-Publication Data is available from the publisher.

This book is an authorized translation of the 2nd German edition published and copyrighted 2007 by Hippokrates Verlag, Stuttgart. Title of the German edition: Praxis der Tuina-Therapie: Atlas zur Behandlung von Erwachsenen und Kindern.

Translator: Sabine Wilms, PhD, Taos, NM, USA

Photos: Yvonne Kranz, Munich, Germany

© 2011 Georg Thieme Verlag,
Rüdigerstrasse 14, 70469 Stuttgart, Germany
http://www.thieme.de
Thieme New York, 333 Seventh Avenue,
New York, NY 10001, USA
http://www.thieme.com

Cover design: Thieme Publishing Group
Typesetting by medionet Ltd., Berlin, Germany
Printed in Italy by L.E.G.O. S.p.A., Vicenza

ISBN 978-3-13-153801-7   1 2 3 4 5 6

Preface to the English Edition

Up to now, I have spent half of my life in my homeland in China and the other half here in Germany. In both my life and my work, I find myself constantly shuttling back and forth between East and West and between their two mentalities. As a physician, I always let myself be guided by two concepts. On the one hand, by a linear concept that is rooted in a logical conclusion based on the application of anatomy-physiology and classic physics in accordance with strictly defined terms and conditions. On the other hand, by a nonlinear concept in which conclusions are drawn on the basis of perception and conviction, supported by quantum physics. When I practice *tuina*, this means that I concern myself not only with solid structures but with processes, movements, and vibrations. All of this together is, after all, "energy." Engaging with this energy, which was already called "*qi*" in ancient China, will be unavoidable for the natural sciences in the future.

The theory of Traditional Chinese Medicine shows that humans must be in harmony with their environment and with themselves if they want to be and remain healthy. This pursuit of harmony is found not only in the linear concept of anatomy but also in the nonlinear concept of energy, of the energy (*qi*) that keeps the whole system together and makes it complete. Energy is the potential of any action. This refers to the potential as the result of which something can happen or change.

The human body possesses a self-healing and self-regulating energy that allows the person to feel healthy. However, if there is a blockage—a disturbance in the movement of the energy—disharmony results. When the blockage is not resolved and the disturbance lasts too long, the patient feels unwell, which can lead to disease. Disturbances can come from the person's environment and from him- or herself, for example political unrest or stressful social influences, but also one's personal lifestyle. *Tuina* practitioners detect these disturbances and attempt to eliminate them by means of their consciousness and concentration through their hands and the application of their own body. To preserve their own inner balance and strengthen their physical energy, *tuina* practitioners in China practice *qigong* on a daily basis.

Both concepts are necessary if we are to embrace the universe and the world around us holistically and hence also understand how to view the patient holistically, for the sake of prevention as well as therapy. This is also where the future lies.

Weizhong Sun

Preface to the Second German Edition

Our intention with this book is to provide easily comprehensible instructions for *tuina* for practitioners of Western medicine. The book is meant to open up accompanying and alternative strategies for practitioners knowledgeable in manual therapy, with a focus on disturbances of the locomotor system. We wish to show complementary treatment options for diseases in the areas of general medicine, internal medicine, gynecology, and pediatrics. In addition, we wish to address physicians, naturopaths, physical therapists and ergotherapists, massage therapists, midwives, and parents.

In this respect, our book takes the familiar Western diagnostic terminology into account and uses generally understood terms in the instructions for self-treatment.

Understanding the theory of Chinese medicine is not an indispensable requirement for learning *tuina* therapy.

This book is the official textbook of the German Tuina Academy. The academy is a center for continuing education and advanced training in medicine with a focus on Traditional Chinese Medicine (TCM). The German Tuina Academy cooperates with the University of TCM in Shandong in an arrangement that is unprecedented in Europe. Training includes both therapeutic and preventative treatments. It presents the entire range of *tuina* therapy rather than, as is often the case in other training centers, only a small part, for example, *tuina* massage.

Additional information can be found at www.tuina-akademie.de.

January 2007
Weizhong Sun
Arne Kapner

Acknowledgements from the Second German Edition

Our thanks go to everybody who helped to complete this book, especially to the patient photographers Yvonne Kranz and Daniela Kühberger, and the no less patient models Salomé, Saphir, and Monika Mayer. Likewise, we are grateful to Barbara Wedell and Dr. Petra von Recklinghausen, MD, for their accurate editing.

In addition, we are grateful for the expert advice of Professor Wang Xin Lu of Shandong TCM University.

Picture Credits

Figs. 8.1, 8.2, 8.3a, 8.3b, 8.4b, 8.5, 8.6, 8.7c, 8.8a, 8.8b, 8.9, 8.10a, 8.10b, 8.11c, 8.12b, 8.13a, 8.14, 8.15b:
From Pape U. Praxis Thai-Massage. Stuttgart: Sonntag; 2009.

Figs. 8.3c, 8.4a, 8.7b, 8.7d, 8.11b, 8.12a:
From Roemer AT. Medical Acupuncture in Pregnancy. Stuttgart–New York: Thieme Publishers; 2005.

Figs. 8.7a, 8.13b, 8.15a:
From Feely R. Yamamoto New Scalp Acupuncture. Principles and Practice. 2nd edition. Stuttgart–New York: Thieme Publishers; 2011.

Fig. 8.11a:
From Strittmatter B. Identifying and Treating Blockages to Healing. Stuttgart–New York: Thieme Publishers; 2003.

Contents

1 Foundations

Development and History

The Chinese term for traditional manual therapy—*tuina*—refers to two of its main techniques, namely *tui* = pushing and pressing, and *na* = grasping and pulling. Nevertheless, for approximately 500 years, *tuina* has served as the umbrella term for a variety of manual treatment forms. The older name used for manual treatments, *an mo*, means, roughly translated, pressing and rubbing. This treatment form has a tradition that is 5000 years old.

The modern term *tuina* summarily refers to pushing and rubbing techniques to regulate the energetic channels, acupressure, and a variety of pressure treatments on channel points and extra points, grasping and stretching techniques, as well as techniques and manipulations to mobilize the joints and spinal column. The system also includes procedures for self-treatment, for example, isometric tension exercises. *Tuina* is applied both therapeutically and preventatively.

Manual forms of therapy (*an mo*) are mentioned for the first time in the *Huang Di Nei Jing* (*Inner Classic of the Yellow Emperor*). This text originated in the last two centuries BCE and contains instructions for treating back pain, facial paralysis, and gastrointestinal disorders.

The first known text to be devoted exclusively to manual therapy appeared between 220 and 265 CE. During this time, the art of manual healing had developed into an independent therapeutic discipline and its application was reserved for practitioners with specialized training. The Tang dynasty (618–907 CE) witnessed the introduction of a system of self-treatment for the treatment and prevention of disease, as well as of instructions for the manual treatment of infants and children. During this Golden Age of Chinese culture, these treatment methods also spread to the neighboring countries of Korea, Japan, and India. During the Song dynasty (Northern Song, 960–1127 CE), manual treatment forms also appeared in the context of obstetrics. Between the 10th and 14th centuries, several different lineages were synthesized into a discipline that advanced during the Ming dynasty (1368–1644 CE) to become a separate academic subject, referred to by the term *tuina* since the 16th century, and taught at the Imperial School of Medicine.

In step with the introduction of Western-style medicine to China, the range of indications for *tuina* treatment has changed. Since 1979, China has had a government-regulated 5-year training program ending in a diploma. There are currently at least 10 universities with *tuina* departments.

Preparations for Treatment

As a general rule, we recommend placing the patient in as comfortable a position as possible. In the supine position, the patient should lie with the head or upper body slightly elevated and the knees slightly flexed, propped up on a cushion or rolled towel. When lying face down, the top of the head should be positioned level or slightly lower. You can place a roll under the bend of the feet to prevent the toes from touching the surface. In patients with severe lumbar lordosis, it is also helpful to place a slightly domed pillow under the belly.

To treat the upper extremities, patients should generally assume a sitting position. Unless it obstructs your movements, you can also use a chair with a backrest for this purpose. The arm to be treated should always be placed in a comfortable position. Relevant advice is found in the instructions below.

The room temperature should be around 20–22°C. In China, patients commonly wear comfortable, light clothing similar to gym- or swimwear. Similar Western-style clothing is acceptable. To make orientation easier for the practitioner, it is advantageous if the part of the body to be treated is not covered with clothing. This can be decided on an individual basis. In all cases, the clothing should preserve the patient's body heat in such a way that the patient will not feel cold during the standard 10 to 40 minutes of treatment at normal room temperature.

For the practitioner, it is important from the outset to optimize the application of force and not to assume overly strenuous positions. This includes a positive attitude toward the patient and the compassion that is necessary for communication to adjust the intensity of the treatment. Setting the height of the sitting surface and treatment table correctly is of primary importance. All tables should have movable head- and footrests attached, and an opening for the face in the headrest is useful. The practitioner should always wear sufficiently roomy clothing that does not restrict his or her range of movement.

The practitioner should have closely clipped nails to prevent scratches and pressure-related injuries. The practitioner must remember to remove any objects that could harm the patient and him- or herself, such as rings, watches, and sharp pieces of clothing (belts, buckles), before any session. The practitioner's hands should be warm and, if necessary, be washed with warm water.

During treatment sessions, the patient should be questioned and observed regarding pain. With the prospect of improvement, most patients will tolerate temporary discomfort; inadequate communication, however, predestines failure.

A gentle approach is of particular importance in the context of obstetrics. If possible, the intensity should be increased only slowly because treatment can lead to vegetative symptoms and cardiovascular irregularities. Accordingly, it is important to watch for paleness, redness of the face, and sleepy facial expressions, and it is also important to question the patient early on about discomfort, nausea, and dizziness.

We suggest, especially in the first treatment, advising the patient that *tuina* therapy can lead to posttreatment pain. Patients should be encouraged to empty their bowels and bladder prior to treatment. Any treatment immediately after a meal should be discouraged; a sufficient interval is approximately 1 hour.

Treatment Principles

According to Chinese tradition, the goal of treatment lies in restoring the functional unity of the person as well as harmony with the environment (universe). The effects of the environment and emotional disturbances are also taken into consideration in both treatment and diagnosis.

There are three principles that describe how the therapy is supposed to affect the organism:

1. **Treatment aims at the comprehensive and holistic regulation of energy in structures that are disturbed in their functional relations.** In a more specific sense, this also includes a structurally disturbed joint to spinal column connection, for example, or a muscular and tendinous structure being restored to its original, natural functional condition.
2. **A therapeutic effect near the focus of the pathology is intended**. The choice of therapeutic measures determines which form of energy is brought close to the disturbed structures. Locally disturbed energies are regulated by means of different forms of manual therapy, for example, acupressure, pushing techniques, or rubbing.
3. **Treatment aims at sending remote signals**. This is related to notions discussed in Western medicine in the context of gate control therapy. What this refers to is a remote treatment that, for example, affects pain and functional disturbances in the internal organs and/or channels from a channel point.

According to Chinese tradition, disturbed health can be caused by negative effects from the environment. In other cases, we can assume internally derived causes (e.g., emotional disturbances). Let us illustrate this with the example of headache:

Any headache that is accompanied by symptoms of repletion (aka fullness) is explained as due to the harmful influence, for example, of cold or warm wind, damp heat, and emotional disturbances (e.g., rage). Treatment aims at removing these harmful influences from the body.

In another example related to headache, symptom combinations that can be categorized as symptoms of vacuity (aka emptiness, deficiency) can be ascribed, for example, to a weakness of blood and lack of vital energy (*qi*). In this case, therapy is intended to build blood and *qi* and to restore their flow.

In this book, we have preceded instructions for treatment with symptom constellations of repletion and vacuity in those cases where experience shows that subjective negative sensations and vegetative symptoms present considerable side-effects in Western understanding as well, such as in cervicocephalic syndrome.

Cold sensations are preferably addressed with therapeutic forms that deliver warmth to the tissue—pressing, rubbing, and acupressure.

Acute complaints should initially be treated near the area of the complaint with an emphasis on the symptoms.

For **chronic complaints**, you should primarily address the cause of the pain. This is illustrated as follows:

Lumbar disk herniation is often accompanied by acute pain in the lower extremities while the lumbar region is barely affected or not at all. In such cases, treatment can initially be concentrated on the symptoms of pain in the lower leg and foot.

In cases of chronified lumbar complaints with recurrent or permanent pain radiating into the lower extremities, you will primarily address the causal complaints in the back and lumbar region and treat the distal symptoms in subsequent treatment steps.

Selection of the treatment form is ultimately based on the effort to balance *yin* and *yang*, repletion and vacuity. The elusive notion of *qi*, a form of energy that is supposed to move in the channels and, depending on symptoms, is either blocked or too concentrated in its velocity, determines the therapeutic approach.

The principles of Chinese medicine also include the need to synchronize the intensity of treatment with the seasons. During spring and summer, when the temperatures are rising, you should limit the use of heat-generating treatment methods as therapies that promote *yang*. With dropping temperatures in the fall and winter, on the other hand, *yang*-supporting treatment forms should be considered more often.

In the choice of treatment, weather conditions are also taken into consideration. According to traditional thinking, persistent hot, humid weather requires a different approach than cold and dry weather.

Age and gender must also be considered in your choice of treatment. Especially in older persons, we recommend a more stimulating approach.

In children, who have a tendency to oscillate quickly between symptoms of repletion and vacuity, we recommend a quick succession of tonifying and detonifying measures in roughly balanced distribution.

Intensity and Duration of *Tuina* Treatment in Cases with Repletion and Vacuity Symptoms

Depending on the symptoms of repletion or vacuity (**Table 1.1**), you should modify pressure and frequency of stimulation within the time interval for each treatment form (e.g., *an*, *tui*, *na*) as well as the duration of treatment as a whole. **Figure 1.1** establishes the relationship between time and intensity. Hereby, the peak of intensity, for example, the application of pressure in the therapeutic form *an*, should be the amount just submaximally bearable for the patient, while the intensity in the flat and

Table 1.1   Summary of symptoms of repletion and vacuity

	Repletion	Vacuity
General condition	Feeling of fullness in the chest and upper abdomen, loud voice	Fatigue, taciturn, quiet voice
Constitution	Normal strength	Tired, thin, lacking strength
Complexion	Normal	Pale
Pain	Localizable, sensitive to pressure	Not localizable precisely, diffuse
Sweating	No/slightly	Yes
Feces	Solid/constipation	Soft
Urine	Scant, dark or concentrated	Plentiful, clear
Tongue	Thick fur	Pale, scant fur
Pulse	Replete, surging	Fine, vacuous

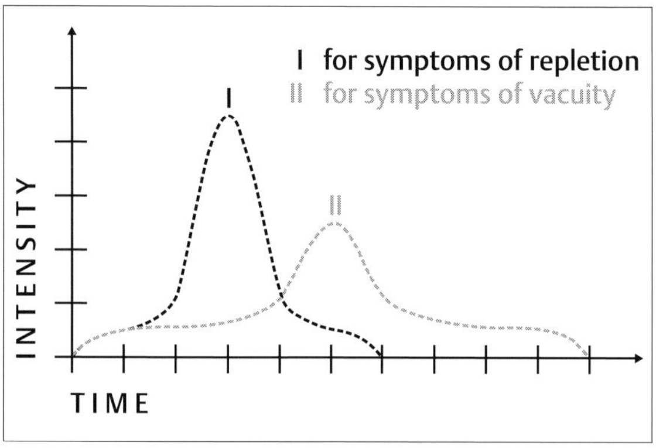

Fig. 1.1

outstretched curve should be roughly half of the bearable intensity.

In cases where symptoms of repletion predominate, you should aim for a shorter time and greater intensity.

In cases with predominant symptoms of vacuity, the intensity (peak clearly lower) should be built up more slowly and then be allowed to drop more slowly as well. When clinical symptoms do not visibly tend toward either repletion or vacuity, you have to find a solution in between these variations.

The same rules that apply for individual treatment forms in accordance with the symptomatic state can also be applied to the course of a treatment session. More intensive stimulations, for example, acupressure, deep transverse friction, deep pushing, or scratching, are associated with the peak zone.

General Instructions for Treatment

All *tuina* techniques require fine synchronization between treatment speed and intensity. This particularly applies to forms of treatment that cover large areas of the body, like pushing.

The best initial contact and feedback on the sensation in the deep tissues is achieved with dry hands on dry skin. It is important, with still bearable pressure intensity, not to leave any skin irritation, even with repeated pushing. When treating clothed body parts (back, proximal sections of the extremities), make sure that the clothes permit pushing, without slipping during pushing.

Pushing is made a lot easier, especially in sections of the extremities that are covered with dense hair, when the practitioner holds a thin smooth towel during pushing. The towel can facilitate traction techniques on the fingers and toes when sweating hands and feet make gripping difficult.

The pertinent literature describes the use of water, oil, or other lubricants. Should you decide to use any in individual cases, we recommend sesame oil. In clinic, talcum powder has proven very useful if the practitioner has moist hands, as well as for patients with very sensitive skin. It especially facilitates the fine rubbing movements on the hands of children and infants. In feverish conditions, briefly wiping the patient down with rubbing alcohol before any *tuina* treatment can be useful, but we do not offer this advice here as a general recommendation.

The Appendix contains charts of the channels, a compilation of recommended acupressure points, and a glossary of *tuina* terminology.

The instructions are generally formulated in such a way that the procedures described under the "General Treatment" sections serve as a framework for the first treatment unit.

The practitioner should then compile a selection of additional treatment forms from the general section, on the basis of questioning the patient at the end of the treatment unit and at the beginning of the subsequent one.

The same guideline applies to the specific treatment recommendations for further planning, even when no general section is listed.

The selection of treatment forms according to symptoms of vacuity or repletion is based on the major disturbances. Not all signs must be present or weighed against each other.

From the third treatment unit on, you should also include pathologic symptoms of the adjacent or more distal regions of the body.

As already mentioned above, the intensity must be adjusted to each patient's initial condition and to feedback after procedures. A substantial increase in complaints at the beginning is rare, but must then be taken as reason to proceed more gently and to increase the intensity and total duration of a treatment unit more slowly. It should also prompt you to test the diagnosis.

If symptoms call for a gradual approach, approximately two to three treatment units per week are suitable. This also applies to chronic conditions.

If a quick succession is more appropriate, 10 treatment units within 4 or 5 weeks serves as a guideline.

Contraindications

General exemptions for *tuina* treatment include fresh wounds, joint and extensive soft-tissue infections, acute gout arthropathy, chronic ulcerations of the skin, lymphangitis, florid tuberculosis infections, septic conditions, and malignant tumors. During pregnancy, the abdominal area and the dorsal and lumbar regions are off limits. By the same token, treatment should not be performed if the patient is greatly exhausted or under the influence of alcohol.

Basic *Tuina* Techniques, Treatment of Adults

Tui 推 **Pushing**

This technique is applied with the thumb tip, with the gripping surface of the thumb's distal phalanx, or more frequently with the heel of the hand, along the channels across muscles and ligaments. Small and narrow areas can also be worked with the radial edge of the thumb's distal phalanx.

When using the gripping surface and tip, the movement direction of the thumb is forward in the direction of the thumb extension. With the radial edge of the thumb (**Fig. 1.2**), push in the lengthwise direction or across the longitudinal axis of the hand in the direction of the other fingers, which can be positioned to provide support.

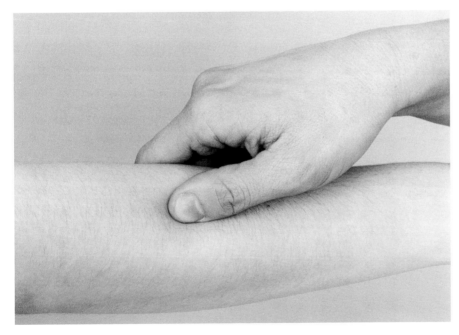

Fig. 1.2

With the ball of the hand, namely the surface of the hand consisting of thenar, hypothenar, and the small area above the proximal row of the carpal bones, push in a longitudinal direction to the hand as well as crosswise to it (**Figs. 1.3** and **1.4**).

The latter pushing direction is well suited to long-distance treatment on top of the channels, in which case the second hand is placed on the back of the first hand to amplify the pressure. *Tui* applied with the ball of the hand allows for a distribution of pressure over a large area. This avoids causing pain in specific points.

In pushing, you should primarily work on the ligaments, tendons, and muscles. The speed is approximately 5 cm per second and can be reduced if necessary.

The non-material vector resulting from pushing and pressing enters the deep tissue at an angle of about 45° inclination to the surface.

The applied force should remain constant and depend on the patient's age, constitution, and the intensity of the complaint manifestation. When in doubt, use restraint in applying force at the beginning of a treatment sequence, especially in the context of the pushing techniques with fist or elbow described below.

Most Chinese authors also describe *tui* by means of the fist, that is, with the knuckles of fingers 2–5 and the associated back sides of the proximal phalanges, to treat larger areas more intensively. This method should preferably be used for patients with thicker subcutaneous fatty tissue on the trunk and larger sections of the extremities.

It is also possible to use the tip of the elbow or the dorso-ulnar side of the lower arm. Depending on how far the joint is flexed, this technique affects a more or less limited treatment surface. To regulate the dosage better in procedures that require stronger pushing, the practitioner should interlock the hands and use the assisting arm to steer the application of force with the treatment arm. You can apply this technique along the thoracic and lumbar spinal column and on the buttocks (**Figs. 1.5** and **1.6**).

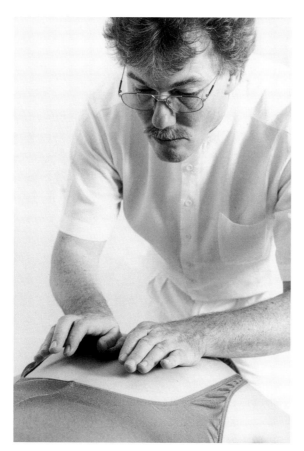

Fig. 1.3

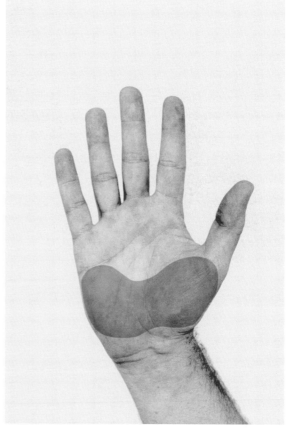

Fig. 1.4

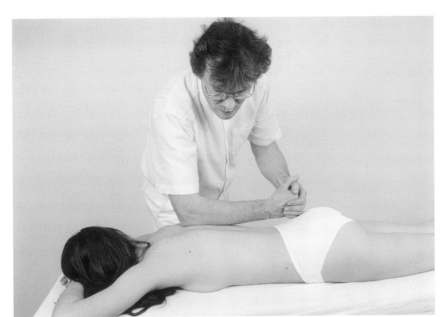

Fig. 1.5

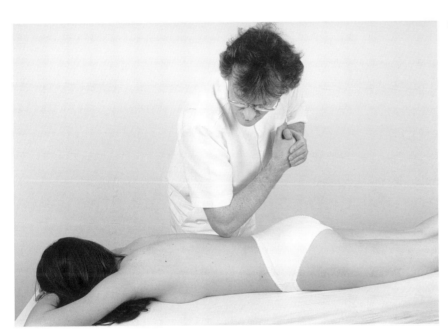

Fig. 1.6

Rou 揉 Kneading

In this technique, executed preferably with the grasping surface of the thumb's distal phalanx and the ball of the hand, pushing is combined with small gyrating movements (circular pushing). The frequency of the circular movements is roughly 60–200 per minute (**Figs. 1.7** and **1.8**).

Avoid causing reddening of the skin by remaining in one place for too long. Circular movements in the clockwise direction are supposed to have a tonifying effect; movements in the opposite direction a sedating effect.

As in *tui*, you can use the fist and the elbow in the *rou* technique as well. The above-mentioned restrictions also apply here.

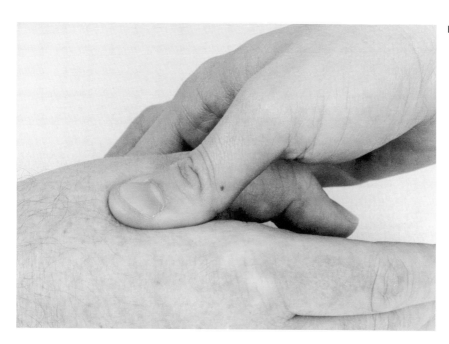

Fig. 1.7

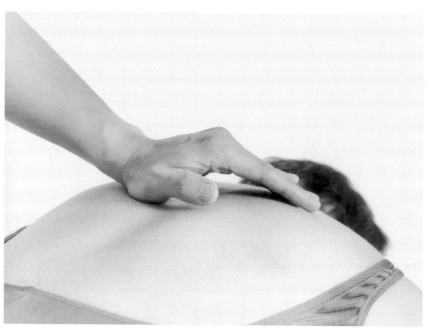

Fig. 1.8

Na 拿 Grasping

The practitioner grasps the skin/subcutaneous region, possibly also the bulge of muscles, with the thumb and index finger or with the thumb and other fingers, pulls it up, then lets it glide through the fingers as if kneading or releases it abruptly.

In each and every case, you should ask the patient whether the grip is tolerable.

Small and tauter areas are grasped between the distal phalanx of the thumb and that of the index finger or the radial side of the middle phalanx of the index finger (**Figs. 1.9** and **1.10**).

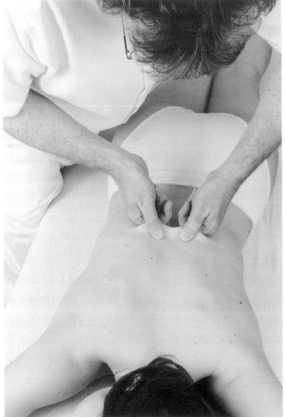

Fig. 1.9

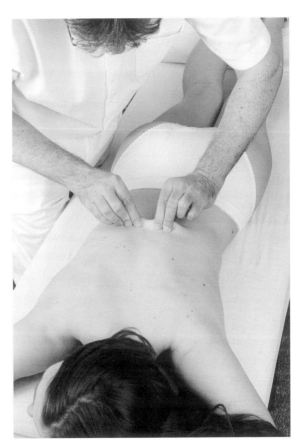

Fig. 1.10

The grip between three and more fingers is suitable for larger volumes. When treating the area of the trapezius muscle, for example, you can also use the fingers, thumb, and thenar (**Fig. 1.11**).

An 按 Pressing

Synonym: Acupressure
Hereby, you apply especially the tip of the thumb, the gripping surface of the thumb, and the tip of the elbow to acupuncture points and areas of the body selected ac-

cordingly. The movement is performed vertically to the surface of the skin, causing even and stable stimulation in the deep layers (**Figs. 1.12** and **1.13**).

You should discuss with the patient whether the slightly stabbing sensation, as in sore muscles, is tolerable.

Increase pressure slowly over 2 or 3 seconds, one to three times in each point, hold for 2 or 3 seconds, and release slowly. This recommendation also applies for all the following variations of acupressure.

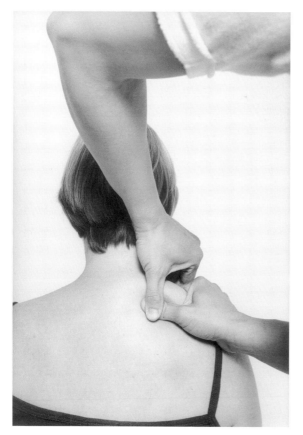

Fig. 1.11

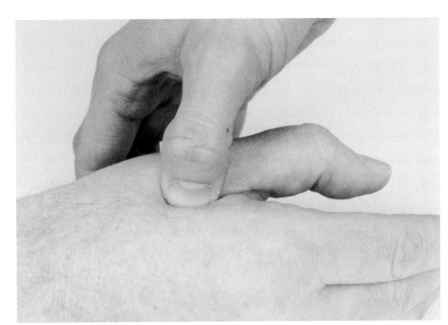

Fig. 1.12

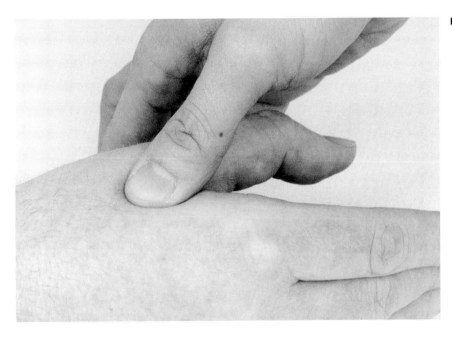

Fig. 1.13

For acupressure with the tip of the elbow, bend the joint 100–120° while the forearm remains in the neutral position between pronation and supination. This technique lends itself particularly well to treatments on top of large cross-sections of muscle, for example, the lumbar region, buttocks, or thighs. The pressure is easily directed when the hand of the treating arm clasps the opposite shoulder, and the upper body is supported on the edge of the treatment table by means of the other arm (**Fig. 1.14**).

If the patient cannot tolerate pressure concentrated in a small area, it can be advantageous especially in slightly concave areas of the body (chest, back, abdomen, and proximal sections of the extremities) to use the palms of the hands or parts of them. Raise the fingers slightly.

We recommend that you utilize both the thenar and the radial edge of the thumb. To better regulate the application of force and clearly increase the effect, position the palm of the second hand on the back side of the thenar and the ulnar side of the thumb and extend the elbow joints (**Fig. 1.15**).

In addition, pressure can be applied with the closed fist via the back sides of the proximal phalanges of fingers 2–5. We recommend limiting this technique to areas with larger amounts of soft tissue, for example, the lumbar region, buttocks, and thighs (**Fig. 1.16**).

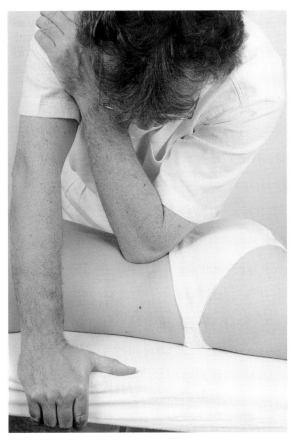

Fig. 1.14

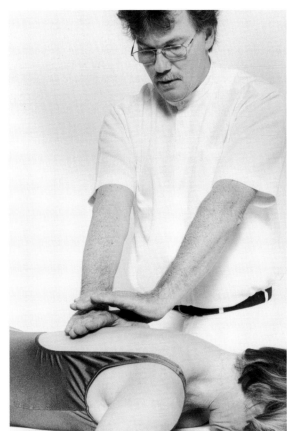

Fig. 1.15

Fig. 1.16

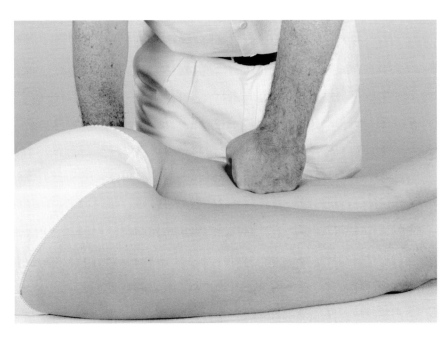

Gun 滚 Rolling

Here, we especially use the distal ulnar edge of the hand and the ulnar side of the proximal joint of the little finger to apply rolling movements (executing the movement between flexion, extension, and rolling) to the treatment area (**Fig. 1.17**).

The practitioner's elbow is flexed slightly. The movement is caused by rapid pronation and supination of the forearm with alternating stretching and bending movements of the wrist (**Fig. 1.18a–c**). Hold the fingers in a functional position (slightly opened hand).

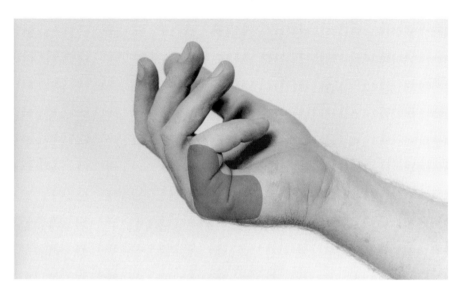

Fig. 1.17

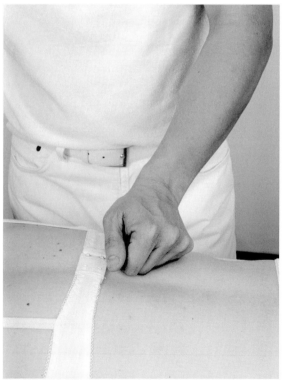

Fig. 1.18a

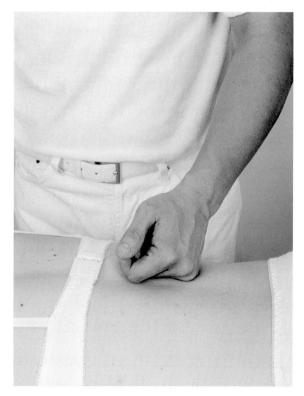

Fig. 1.18b

The rolling axis runs across the back sides of the three ulnar proximal joints of the fingers (3–5). When rolling off, the ulnar edge of the hand, the distal section of the back of the hand, and the back sides of the proximal phalanges of fingers 3 and 4 are placed in the direction of the back of the hand. During the opposite movement toward the palm of the hand, the ulnar edge of the little finger and the distal ulnar edge of the metacarpus remain in contact with the surface.

Movements are performed progressively in the direction of the specified sequence or of the main expanse of the specified area. The goal is to produce a mild but deep stimulation in the muscles.

The *gun* technique is particularly suitable for the treatment of paresthesia and the primary therapy of painful contractions. It is also used for more intensive local treatments, for example, in epicondylitis and on top of the recess of the knee joint with extended treatment time (10–20 minutes).

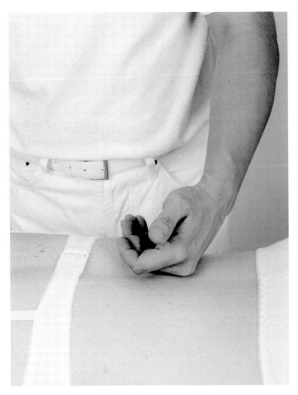

Fig. 1.18c

Rolling across the ulnar edge of the distal phalanx of the little finger lends itself to being applied on small areas: with the thumb extended and the other fingers flexed (loosely closed fist), the forearm moves by turning rapidly (pronation and supination).

A more spacious rolling movement is performed with a closed fist via the back side of the proximal phalanges and the proximal and middle joints of fingers 2–5, by rapidly flexing and extending the wrist (**Fig. 1.19a, b**).

Rocking movements of the wrist radially and ulnarly, that is, transverse to the rolling-off direction, are possible as well.

We consider the above-mentioned techniques by means of the edge of the thumb and ulnar edge of the hand more workable.

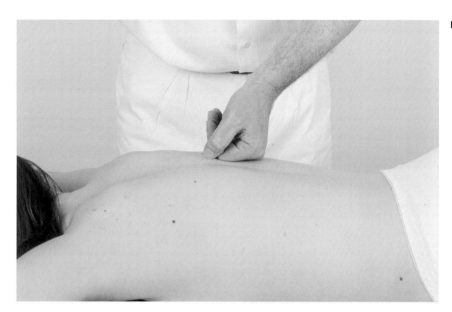

Fig. 1.19a

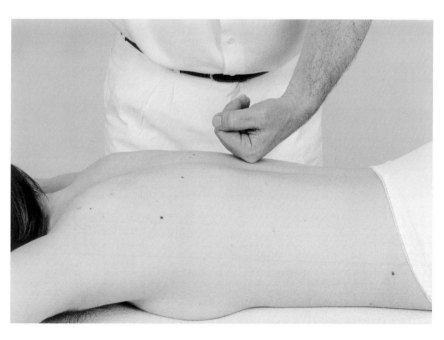

Fig. 1.19b

2 Disorders of the Locomotor System: Specific Techniques

Spinal Column

■ Cervical Spinal Column

Symptoms of Vacuity

Neck pain, dizziness, and seeing stars when sitting up or standing up, noise in the ears, reduced hearing, moist palms of the hands and feet, problems sleeping through the night, irritability, back pain that resembles sore muscles, feeling of weakness in the legs, red tongue without fur, fine rapid pulse.

Symptoms of Repletion

Neck pain radiating into the shoulders and thoracic spinal column area, stabbing pain, easily localized pain, lusterless fingernails, dry skin with diffuse itching, spotty dark red tongue, fine tight pulse.

Cervical Syndrome

Pain associated with the cervical spine as a functional unit, chronic muscle pain, complaints related to the intervertebral disks with or without symptoms of radicular irritation and slipped disks.

For Symptoms of Vacuity

- BL-23
- KI-3

For Symptoms of Repletion

- ST-36, ST-40
- GB-34

General Treatment

An 按 **Pressing**

- With the thumb
- GB-20, GB-12, GB-21
- SI-14, SI-11, SI-10
- LI-14, LI-11

Tui 推 **Pushing**

- With the ball of the hand
- In prone position
- Slowly on top of the bladder channel from the lower section of the cervical spine to the foot, on both sides
- Five to eight times
- Also with the patient seated with pushes from the lower cervical spine to the sacrum

→ **Fig. 2.1**

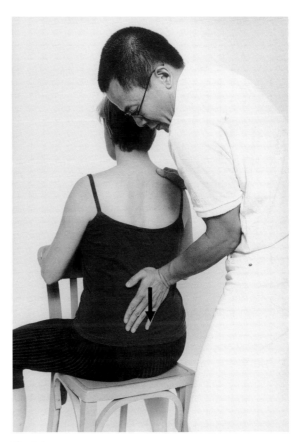

Fig. 2.1

Na 拿 Grasping

- In prone position
- With interlocked fingers, grasp the neck muscles between the balls of the hand and push toward each other, then pull toward the ceiling.
- Increase the pull slowly, hold for 1–2 seconds, and let go without completely releasing the grip.
- Three to five times
→ **Fig. 2.2**

Rou 揉 Kneading

- With the thumb or the tip of the thumb
- On the seated patient
- Place your free hand on the patient's forehead. With the gripping surface of the thumb, perform circling movements with gentle pressure on top of the bladder and gallbladder channels, descending from the back of the head across the neck.
- Patient feedback should reveal particularly sensitive areas.
- Treat both sides, limiting treatment to the paravertebral region.
- About 3 minutes
→ **Fig. 2.3**

Gun 滚 Rolling

- With the ulnar edge of the hand
- Starting from medial across the dispersion area of the horizontal branch of the trapezius, on both sides
- Three minutes
→ **Fig. 2.4**

or

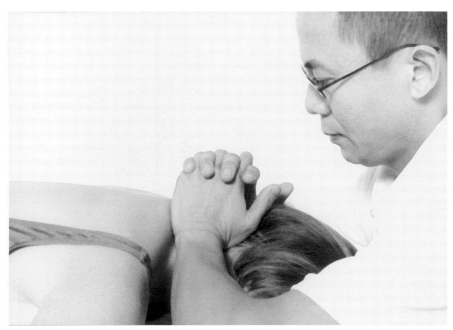

Fig. 2.2

Rou 揉 Kneading

- With the thumb or ball of the hand
- The previously described treatment can also be continued with this technique on the area of the horizontal trapezius on both sides.
- Three minutes

→ **Fig. 2.4**

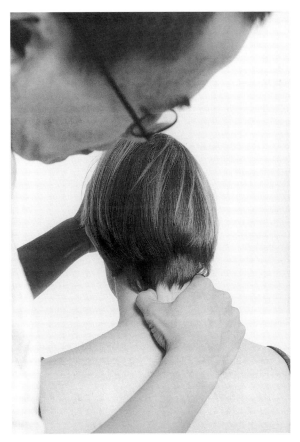

Fig. 2.3

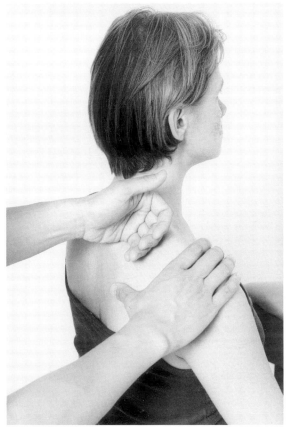

Fig. 2.4

Gun 滚 **Rolling**

- With the ulnar edge of the hand
- On the seated patient
- Treat the three channels on the *yang* side of the arm, ascending from the middle of the forearm up to the shoulder, on both sides.
- Three to five passes
→ **Fig. 2.5**

Qian Yin 牵引 **Traction**

- On the seated patient with the arm raised 45° forward and 45° to the side
- Clasp the patient's metacarpus and carpus in both hands. The patient's trunk, which is supported from behind by the chair, serves as the "counterfort".
- Hold the pull for about 10–15 seconds.
- Five to eight times
→ **Fig. 2.6**

! You can also apply traction by clasping the ring and little finger with both of your corresponding fingers.

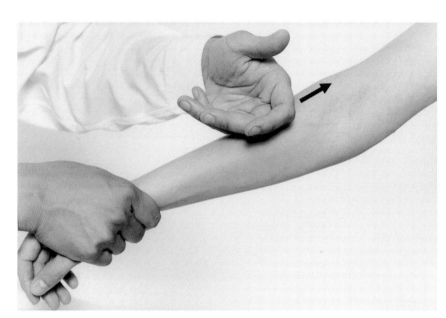

Fig. 2.5

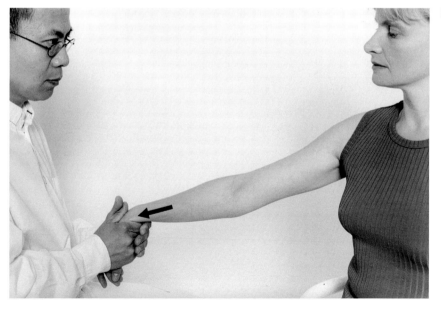

Fig. 2.6

Myogeloses

Painful Rope-shaped Hardenings in the Muscle

Heng Bo 横拨 **Transverse Frictions**

- With the tip of the thumb
- On the seated patient, on top of the paravertebral muscles of the cervical spine
- In quick succession, perform two to three frictions transverse to the path of the muscles.
- You should treat a maximum of two to three muscle hardenings in a row.

→ See **Fig. 2.3**

Knotty Hardenings in the Muscle

Rou 揉 **Kneading**

- With the thumb
- On the seated patient, on top of the paravertebral muscles of the cervical spine
- Five to 20 seconds on the affected location

→ See **Fig. 2.3**

! In cases where the technique is experienced as too painful, we recommend localized treatment with the *gun* technique.

Cervicocephalic and Cervicobrachial Syndrome

➡ The section on the "Upper Extremities" (p. 46 ff) contains information on complementary treatment techniques.

Qian Yin 牵引 **Traction**

- With the patient seated on a stool
- The practitioner sits elevated on the treatment table, behind the patient, bends the legs, and supports the forefoot on the edge of the stool. With the balls of the thumbs, grip the back of the patient's head medial to the mastoid, on both sides. The fingers are pointing cranially and lie flat against the back and side of the head. The bent elbows immobilize the patient in front of the shoulder on both sides. The traction movement is achieved by straightening the patient's cervical spine (reducing the kyphosis) and shifting your trunk backward.
- The patient then relaxes and leans backward while also being supported at the back between your thighs. Do not allow the patient's cervical spine to sink into an increasing kyphosis and do not release your grip on the back of the head.
- The traction treatment is performed about two times in a row as a continuous pull for 5–10 seconds each. If the patient can tolerate the therapy, you can apply a short increased pull on the previously held tension by straightening your spinal column.

→ **Fig. 2.7**

Fig. 2.7

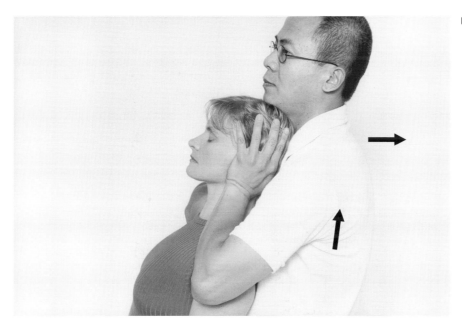

Xuan Zhuan Qian Yin 旋转牵引 **Rotating Traction**

Manipulation of the Cervical Spine
• In supine position
• The cervical spine and the upper part of the shoulders extend beyond the upper edge of the table. Guide and support the patient's head and cervical spine.
• The neck lies in your hand, your thumb is abducted. Avoid gripping the cervical spine too firmly (pinching). The second hand supports the traction by lying flat against the chin and steering the rotation. To test mobility, rotate in both directions as far as the patient's symptoms permit.
→ **Fig. 2.8a**

! For better control in the application of force, immobilize the patient's vertex against your chest and create the traction by shifting your upper body backward and forward.

• In the painful rotation direction, rotate only so far that the patient just begins to feel pain. Ask the patient about discomfort. In all cases, we recommend performing a test pull under rotation and traction.
• Stronger traction results when you prop up your shins against the upper edge of the table, thereby forming a "counterfort" for the traction on the top of the shoulders.
• If the tension held so far does not cause an increase in pain, you can continue with a brief pulling impulse.
• Total length of treatment about 1 minute
→ **Fig. 2.8b**

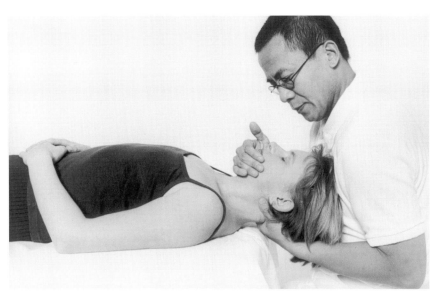

Fig. 2.8a

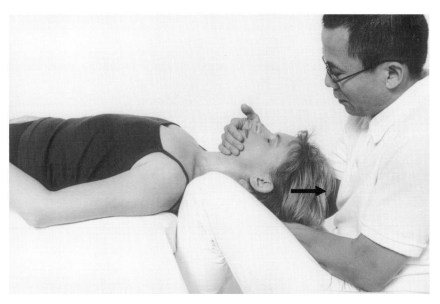

Fig. 2.8b

! In all cases we recommend observing the standard contraindications (Chapter 1, p. 6). If acute symptoms resulting from a proven or suspected slipped disk are present, any manipulative impulse must be avoided.

Xuan Zhuan Fa 旋转法 **Rotating Mobilization of the Cervical Spine**

- In prone position
- Stand in front of the head of the table (e.g., with rotation to the right). Place your left thenar eminence and thumb flat against the upper edge of the patient's scapula. Now grasp the upward-pointing right side of the back of the patient's head from caudal with the other hand. A stretch results on the right levator scapulae and on the opposing paracervical muscles.
- Perform two to three slowly turning rotations, whereby the rotational component and the traction component cover only a short distance. You can follow up with a manipulative impulse.

→ **Fig. 2.9**

! In all cases we recommend observing the standard contraindications (Chapter 1, p. 6). If acute symptoms resulting from a proven or suspected slipped disk are present, any manipulative impulse must be avoided.

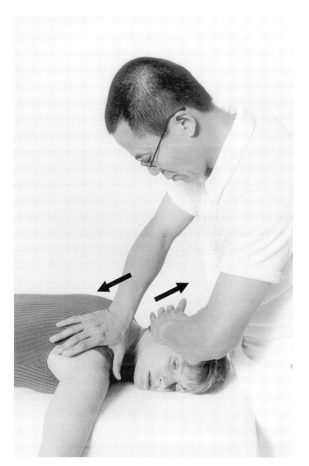

Fig. 2.9

Ce Ban 侧扳 Stretching

- In supine position on the sternocleidomastoid and the scalene muscles (e.g., on the left)
- Stand in front of the head of the table. Place your right hand with the thumb abducted below the patient's neck (do not pinch). The palm of your left hand lies on the top of the patient's shoulder, medial to the acromion. Now bend the patient's head without rotation to the right side.
- Build the stretch slowly and perform two to three rhythmic stretches from a mild initial stretch; hold for 2–3 seconds.

→ **Fig. 2.10**

> **!** In all cases we recommend observing the standard contraindications (Chapter 1, p. 6). If acute symptoms resulting from a proven or suspected slipped disk are present, any manipulative impulse must be avoided.

Xuan Zhuan Fa 旋转法 Rotating Mobilization

- In supine position, stretching the anterior neck muscles (e.g., on the left)
- Rotate the cervical spine to the right. If a thorough rotation is painful or not possible for other reasons, cushion and lift the contact side with a pillow or towel. Place the palm of your left hand flat against the patient's left jaw angle and apply a rotating push cranially and to the right. The right hand lies on the front of the shoulder and on the acromion.
- Two to three stretches from a mild initial stretch

→ **Fig. 2.11**

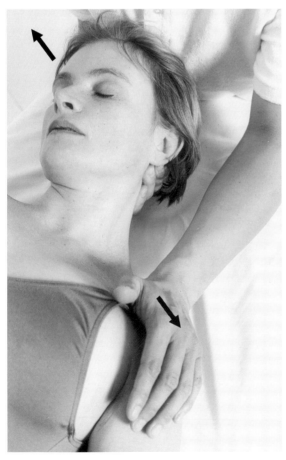

Fig. 2.10

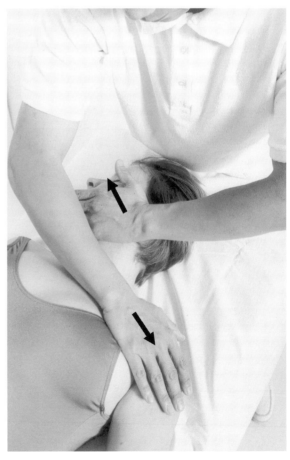

Fig. 2.11

Qian Yin 牽引 **Traction**

- Traction of the five fingers on the side affected by radiating pain. The arm is extended in the elbow and wrist joint, raised approximately 45° to the front and side. With one hand, immobilize the distal forearm. With the two or three ulnar fingers of the other hand, clasp one finger and gradually build the pull through the finger, metacarpus, and wrist; hold for 2–3 seconds, and release.
- Once per finger

→ **Fig. 2.12a, b**

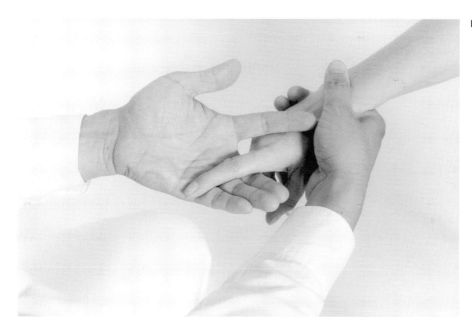

Fig. 2.12a

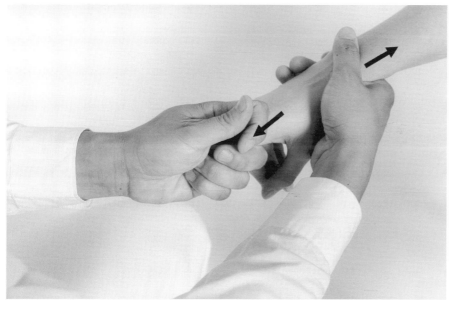

Fig. 2.12b

Qian Yin 牵引 **Traction with Swinging Technique on the Forearm**

- On the seated patient
- Seat yourself to the side and front of the patient and immobilize the top of the patient's shoulder with the hand that is closer to the patient. With the other hand, clasp the metacarpus. In the starting position, the wrist and elbow joints are flexed almost to the maximum, the arm is raised approximately 45° to the front and side.
- Now extend the wrist and elbow joints with a slight inward rotation and momentum and perform a short jerky pull in the final position.
- Five to 10 times

→ **Fig. 2.13a, b**

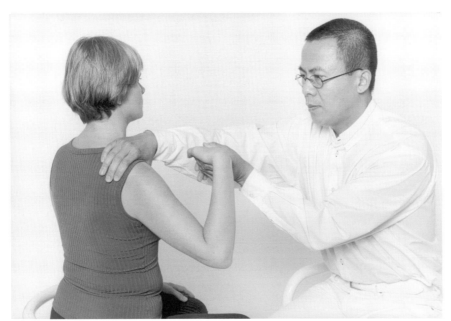

Fig. 2.13a

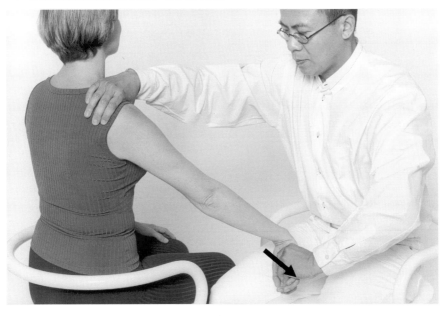

Fig. 2.13b

■ Thoracic and Lumbar Spine

Symptoms of Vacuity

Diffuse pain, localized cold sensation, warmth or pressure are experienced as comfortable, inner disquietude, sleeplessness, damp hands and feet, night sweating, dark red tongue with white fur, fine and rapid pulse.

Symptoms of Repletion

Strong, easily localizable pain, mild everyday movement relieves the pain, dizziness and feeling of heaviness in the head, dark red tongue with yellow fur, stringlike and slippery pulse.

Dorsal, Lumbar, and Sacroiliac Syndrome

Pain that is associated with the back as a functional unit, chronic muscle pain, complaints related to the intervertebral disks with or without symptoms of radicular irritation and slipped disks.

For Symptoms of Vacuity

An 按 **Pressing**

- KI-3
- BL-60

For Symptoms of Repletion

An 按 **Pressing**

- SP-6
- GB-34

General Treatment

An 按 **Pressing**

- BL-23
- BL-40

An 按 **Pressing**

- In prone position
- Place the thenar eminence and thumb broadly on top of the bladder channel, section by section successively in a row caudally. Place the second hand on top of the radial back of the first hand and back of the thumb. Measure the pressure carefully.
- With elbow joints in maximum extension and locked shoulder girdle, stand to the side of the table and con-

trol the pressure by shifting the weight of your body (forward and backward).
- Ask the patient if he or she is tolerating the pressure. Slowly build pressure and then release it, each section once, up to three passes from the upper cervical spine to the sacrum.

→ **Fig. 2.14a, b**

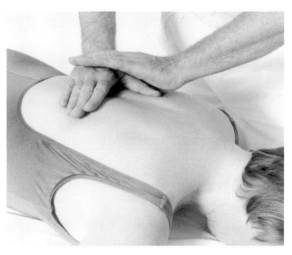

Fig. 2.14a

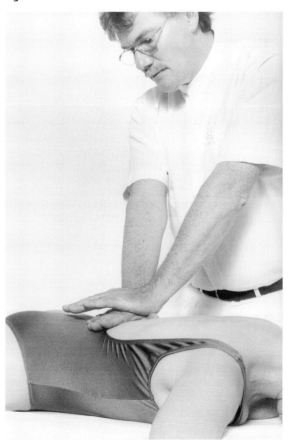

Fig. 2.14b

An 按 **Pressing**

- In prone position
- Stand in front of the head of the table, place the gripping surfaces of the thumbs on SI-14, and support the splayed fingers on both sides loosely on the shoulder blades.
- Slowly increase the pressure and then release it.
- Three to five times
- → **Fig. 2.15**

An 按 **Pressing**

- In prone position; treatment of the eye points on both sides of the back. The so-called eye points of the back are located on the bladder channel below BL-52, at the height of L3 on both sides of the spinal column.
- Stand at the level of the lower section of the lumbar spinal column. With the thumbs, apply pressure to the tissue bilaterally at the level of the transverse process of L3.
- The pressure runs diagonally medially to the plumb line of the body toward the tip of the transverse process of L3. Slowly increase the pressure and then release it.
- Three to five times
- → **Fig. 2.16**

- In one variation, treat the back with kneading movements and alternating pressure with the thumbs and index fingers placed on top of each other in a pinch grip.
- One to 2 minutes

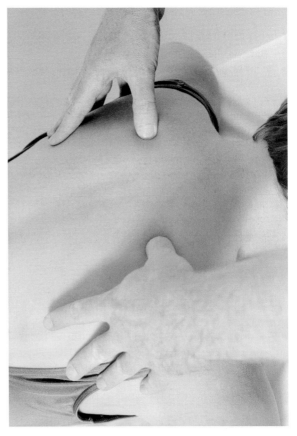

Fig. 2.15

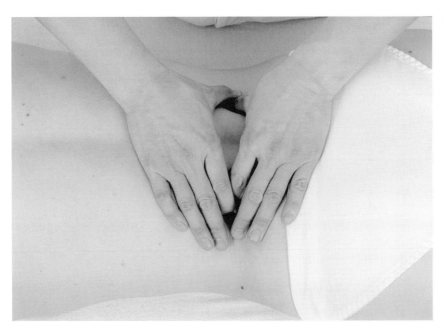

Fig. 2.16

An 按 **Pressing**

- With the elbow
- In prone position; treatment of the eye points on both sides of the back
- Stand to the side of the patient on the side with fewer complaints, bend over far across the back and place the tip of the elbow on top of the bladder channel below the point BL-52. The pressure of the elbow tip runs with a slight medial inclination toward the tip of the transverse process of L3. Holding on to the edge of the table with your free hand, regulate the pressure of the applied elbow tip by balancing the weight of your upper body.

→ **Fig. 2.17**

Pai 拍 **Patting**

- With cupped hands or with the ulnar edges of the hands, with splayed fingers
- In prone position on the paravertebral muscles and the adjacent parts of the thorax and lumbar region
- About 1 minute

→ **Fig. 2.18**

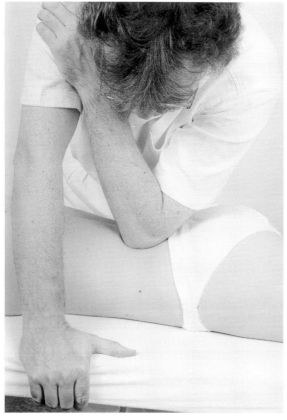

Fig. 2.17

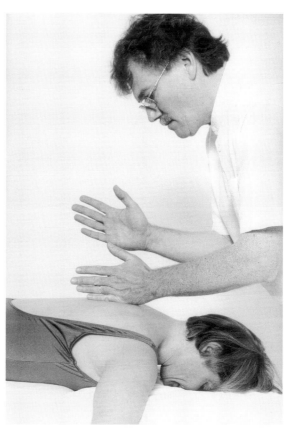

Fig. 2.18

Tui 推 **Pushing**

- In prone position
- Stand by the long side of the table. With the broadly placed ball of the right hand, covered and assisted by the left hand, apply a hard push on the bladder channel from the cervical or thoracic spine down caudally. Hereby, you can also utilize the above-mentioned support technique (see "Basic *Tuina* Techniques" in Chapter 1) in the shoulder girdle, with the upper arms against the upper body and elbow supported on top of the iliac crest.
- Now stroke the bladder channel from the neck to the sacrum and then down from the buttocks across the back of the thighs and lower leg to the lateral edge of the little toe. From the hamstring on down, treat with the thumb-pushing technique. We recommend applying slightly less pressure in the areas of the neck and cervical spine.
- Five times
→ **Fig. 2.19a–d**

> **!** It is important to apply this push without long pauses. Because of the long distance covered by the treatment, this requires some practice. Begin treating the side with the main complaints, for example, the right side. In all cases, treat the parallel-running bladder channel (in the present example then the left side) in the same way. For this purpose, stand on the left side of the patient's body and apply the ball of the left hand.

Rou 揉 **Kneading**

- With the ball of the hand
- In prone position
→ See **Fig. 1.8** in Chapter 1

or

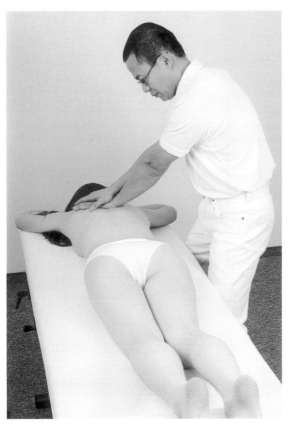

Fig. 2.19a

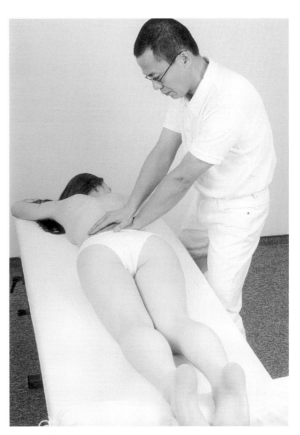

Fig. 2.19b

Gun 滚 **Rolling**

- Across the ulnar edge of the hand
- On the bladder channel, descending to the sacroiliac joint
- Treat both sides, beginning with the side with the main complaints.
- Three to 5 minutes
→ See **Fig. 1.17a–c** in Chapter 1

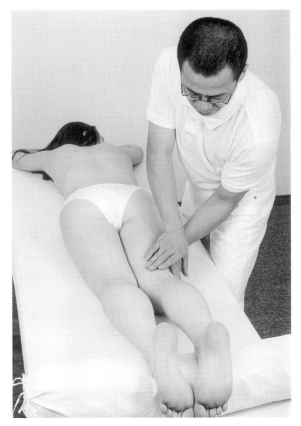

Fig. 2.19c

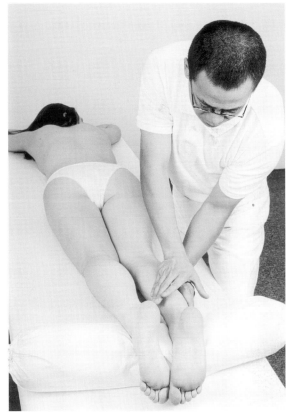

Fig. 2.19d

Dorsal and Dorsolumbar Syndromes

Rou 揉 **Kneading**

- With the thumb
- Seek out particularly sensitive points with the tip of the finger or thumb. They are located primarily by the bladder channel and by the trigger points, also known from Western manual medicine, in the paravertebral area.
- If possible, establish particularly deep contact, slowly build pressure, and then release, up to three times per point.

Zhang Ban Fa 掌扳 **Tangential Counterpush**

In the Area of the Thoracic Spine
- With the ball of the hand
- In prone position
- Stand by the side of the table. Place your hands parallel but facing in opposite directions bilaterally on top of the paravertebral muscles of the thoracic spine. The balls of the hands make firm contact and carry out a pushing movement in opposite directions by means of a short jerking adduction in the shoulder joints.
- Instruct the patient to perform slow breathing movements. During the exhalatory phase, repeat these

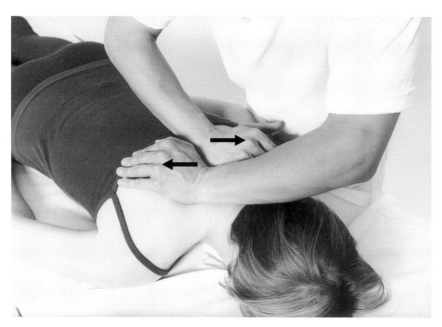

Fig. 2.20a

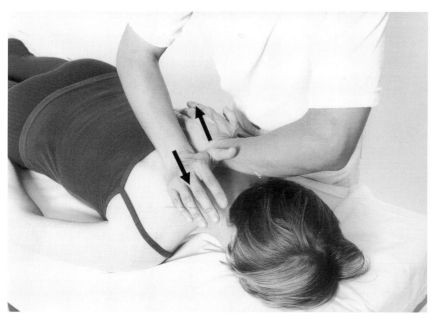

Fig. 2.20b

opposing pushes in quick succession, moving by the width of the ball of the hand from the upper to the lower part of the thoracic spine. Afterward, switch treatment side (right/left) and again repeat the procedure in the descending direction (distally); up to two passes.

→ **Fig. 2.20a, b**

Xuan Zhuan Fa 旋转法 **Rotating Mobilization**

General Technique for Mobilizing the Spinal Column, Primarily for the Thoracic and Lumbar Spine

- Have an additional person immobilize the sitting patient at the thigh with the hands and lateral counterpressure with the knee. The practitioner stands to the side and behind the patient.
- Turn the patient's trunk to the right, for instance. Pass your right arm under the patient's armpit while the

patient's upper arm lies loosely on top of your elbow. Holding the patient as described, perform clockwise movements toward the right, first with a smaller, then with a larger radius. In small movements, the imagined top of the circular movement lies in the lower thoracic spine; in circles with a larger radius, it moves to the area of the sacrum. The patient's ischium should not leave the seating surface. Also avoid rough swinging movements in the pelvis.

- Repeat this technique, circling on the right or left, two to five times.

→ **Fig. 2.21a, b**

 Always begin with small circling movements and increase the radius gradually, depending on the state of the patient's complaints.

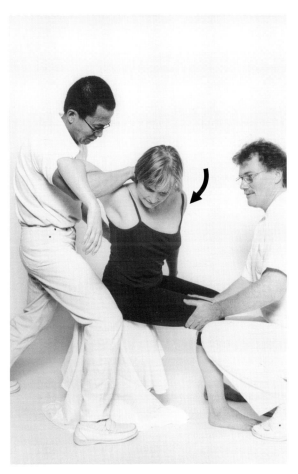

Fig. 2.21a

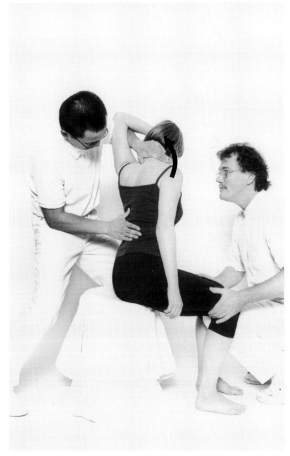

Fig. 2.21b

Fan Gong 反功 Turning Technique

Mobilization of the Dorsolumbar Transition
- In prone position
- This technique is particularly well-suited for the rotating mobilization of the lower dorsal sections and the dorsolumbar transition. When raising one shoulder from this position, the technique additionally increases the patient's lordotic curvature. Sensitivity to curving the thoracic and lumbar spine can limit this technique. You should achieve, for example, a rightward rotation, that is, a rotation in the clockwise direction.
- For this purpose, immobilize the patient's right shoulder with your left hand. Your right hand, placed caudally, provides resistance by the bulge of the right psoas muscle. With your left hand, pull the right shoulder up dorsally and rotate the trunk, one or two times.
→ **Fig. 2.22a, b**

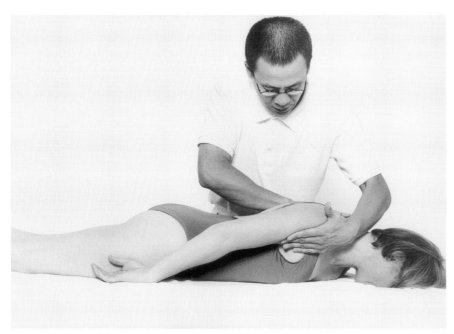

Fig. 2.22a

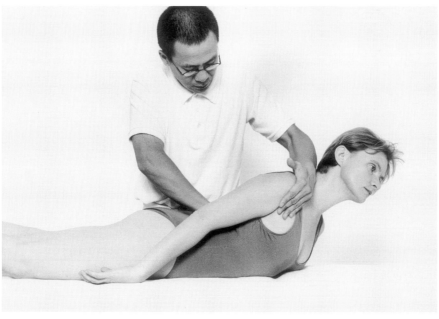

Fig. 2.22b

Lumbosacral Syndrome

Ce Ban 侧扳 **Stretching of the Lumbar Spine**

As a General Mobilization Technique
- In lateral position
- Orienting yourself by the rotational direction of the upper body or the descending rotated segments, perform a rotation toward the right, that is, clockwise when viewed from the cranial direction. Hereby, the patient is lying on the right side of the body. Upper body, abdomen, and lower legs lie near the edge of the table. The leg on top is flexed in the hip and knee, the dorsum of the foot is placed in the back of the knee of the lower leg. The right forearm or the hand of the patient is placed under the head. The patient's left hand lies on the upper abdomen or the top of the chest, the arm is bent and lies flat against the side.
- Immobilize the patient with the inside of the forearm against the lateral wall of the upper chest. Coming from a caudal direction, lay the treatment arm down, with the ball of the hand against the bulge of the distal left paravertebral lumbar muscles and with the inside of the distal forearm on top of the left sacrum and buttocks. Now perform the rotation and stretch on the lower half of the body.
- Once
→ **Fig. 2.23**

 Always check the patient's sensitivity toward rotations carefully before any manipulating impulse.

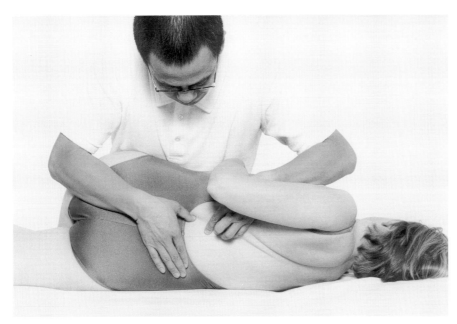

Fig. 2.23

La Tui Fa 拉推法 **Pulling and Pushing**

Rotating Mobilization of the Thoracic and Lumbar Spinal Column, Extension of the Sacroiliac joint, Stretch of the Gluteal Muscles

- In supine position
- This technique is intended to achieve, for example, a rightward rotation of the thoracic spine, the dorsolumbar transition, and the lumbar spine, as well as a dorsal extension of the sacroiliac joint.
- In this case, position yourself on the patient's right side. With your right hand, from the caudal direction take hold of the patient's right leg, flexed in the hip and knee, by the tibial plateau and the knee while grasping the hand of the left extended arm with your right hand. Now slowly apply a pull to cause the rota- tion, transmitted via the shoulder and by forced strad- dling of the flexed hip and lifting the right side of the pelvis (rotation to the left), up to three times.
- The rotation is performed in both directions.
→ **Fig. 2.24**

Treatment variation:
- The patient remains in supine position with arms flat against the body.
- Eliminate the rotation of the thoracic and lumbar spine.
- Slowly flex the knee and hip, alternating between the right and left side, initially only in a hingelike motion toward the ipsilateral shoulder, then by moving the knee in a gradually increasing inward hip rotation toward the sternum and opposite shoulder.
- Five times per side

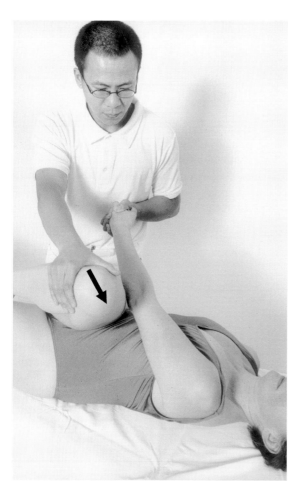

Fig. 2.24

An Xi Ti Tun Fa 按膝提臀法 **Knee–Buttocks Counterpressure and Circular Movement**

Primarily Rotating Mobilization of the Lumbar Spine and Stretch of the Gluteal Muscles

- In supine position with arms placed laterally on the table and the knees and hip in maximum flexion
- With your hand and forearm, immobilize the front sides of the upward-pointing ridges of the shinbones. Your other arm and forearm immobilize the buttocks in a wide embrace. Fixate (lock) your forearms against the trunk.
- The movement is caused by the practitioner by moving the legs and pelvis. The resulting circling movement on the patient points with the apex toward the area of the central and lower lumbar spine, toward the right and left.
- Approximately 1 minute
→ **Fig. 2.25**

 As a general rule, generate only small circling movements.

- To stretch the gluteus minimus, you can subsequently exert a straight push with your forearm onto the upper end of the shinbone, while pulling up the other forearm that is immobilizing the patient's buttocks.

Fig. 2.25

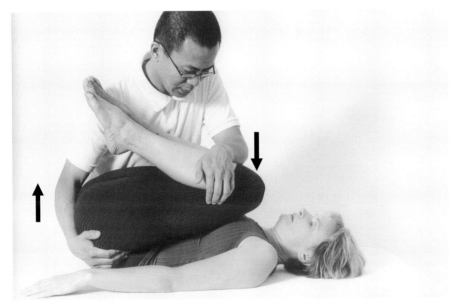

Pain Associated with Lumbago

Piriformis Syndrome, Pseudoradicular Complaints in the Lower Extremities

An 按 **Pressing**

- With the elbow
- In prone position
- GB-30

An 按 **Pressing**

- With the elbow
- In lateral position with flexed hip and knee joints
- GB-29
- → **Fig. 2.26**

An Ban Fa 按扳法 Pressing and Twisting

Mobilization of the Sacroiliac Joint, Stretch of the Quadriceps

- In prone position
- This technique is meant to mobilize the right sacroiliac joint (ventralizing effect on the upper dorsal pole of the sacrum and relative dorsalization of the upper pole of the sacrum).
- The right border of the sacrum is immobilized broadly with the ball of the hand. The fingers lie lightly on the medial right half of the buttocks. Pass your right arm from medial direction beneath the patient's right knee. Place your hand on the back side and outside of the proximal thigh. Position your forearm laterally on the middle section of the thigh, with the patient's knee extending slightly beyond your elbow, so that the distal part of the quadriceps lies in the crook of the arm.

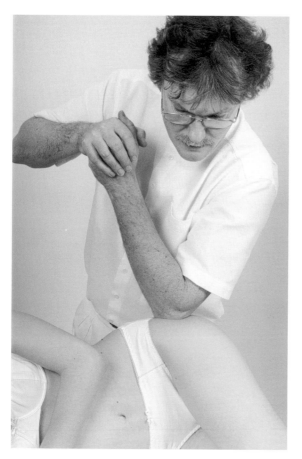

Fig. 2.26

Now perform circling movements with the patient's right leg, with the circle's apex in the right small pelvis. In the greatest extension in the hip joint, the pelvis should rise up slightly from the table.

- When you are standing on the right side, the circling movements are performed in a counterclockwise direction, with an obvious extension component. On the left side, reverse the direction accordingly to clockwise.
- Three to five times

→ **Fig. 2.27**

 Before any manipulation—impulse with adduction in hip joint extension—in all cases we recommend performing a test pull, as is common in manual medicine.

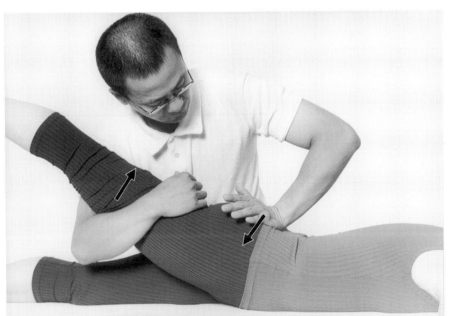

Fig. 2.27

Qian Yin **Traction of the Ischiocrural and Calf Muscles**

- In supine position
- Position yourself by the foot of the table, looking at the head of the table. Stretch the patient's leg in the knee, lift it passively as far as possible, and place the calf in front of your shoulder.
- The hands with interlocked fingers offer resistance by the distal thigh. The patient's ankle joint initially remains extended.
- Keep your trunk upright. The increase and decrease in tension is caused by moving the trunk forward and backward, which arises exclusively from bending and stretching the hip, knee, and ankle joints.

- Three to five times on both sides
→ **Fig. 2.28a–c**

- With sufficient tolerance, you can vary the method by slowly increasing tension with inward and outward rotations as well as by forcibly stretching the calf muscles via the ankle joint, up to three rotations per direction.

! Sensitivity to rotations in the ankle joint can create considerable limitations for this method.

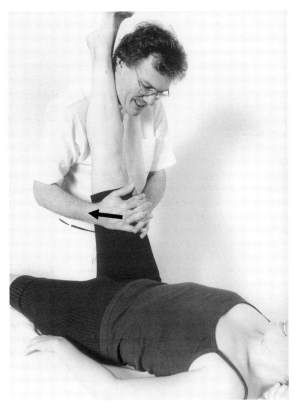

Fig. 2.28a

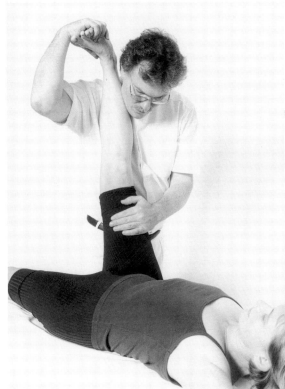

Fig. 2.28b

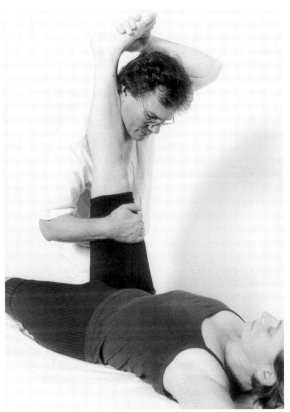

Fig. 2.28c

Qian La Fa 牽拉法   **Traction and Pulling**

- In supine position
- The patient holds on to the upper edge of the table with both hands.
- When treating the right side, position yourself by the foot of the table to the right side, facing the patient and the head of the table. The patient's leg is extended (at the knee) and is raised approximately 30° off the

table. Firmly clamp the ankle area and the back of the foot between your armpit, the inside of the upper arm, and the side of the trunk, and pull. Clasp the patient's lower leg with your hands.

- Place your left leg forward and bend your knees slightly. Keep the trunk upright and slightly backward. First perform a stretch. Maintain this. Now have your right hand, while continuously pulling, glide down to the ankle area and grasp this. At the same time, the left

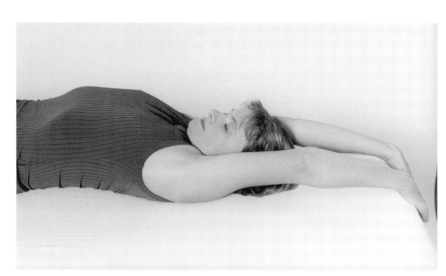

Fig. 2.29a

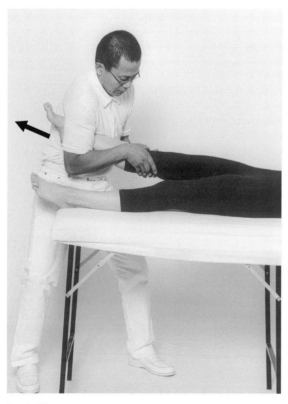

Fig. 2.29b

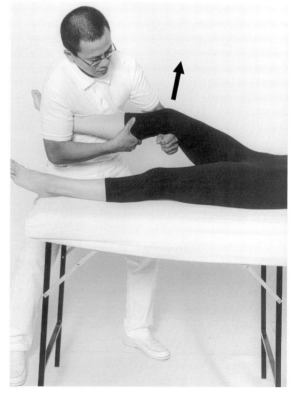

Fig. 2.29c

hand grips and raises the distal section of the thigh off the table. While maintaining the traction in the ankle and foot, increase flexion in the knee as far as possible.

- In the final phase, your left hand leaves its position on the back of the thigh, and the distal left forearm adds yet more flexion-increasing pressure from frontal onto the shin.
- Now free, your left hand also grips the ankle in a rapid movement. Pull again on the leg with a jerk, two to three times.

→ **Fig. 2.29a–f**

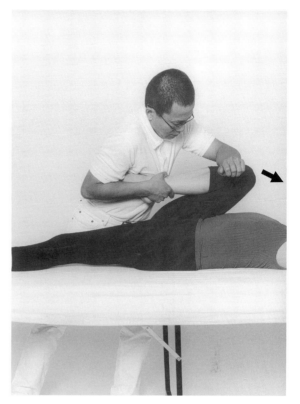

Fig. 2.29d

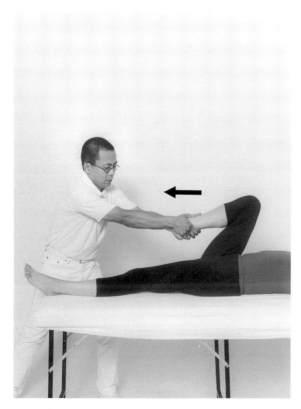

Fig. 2.29e

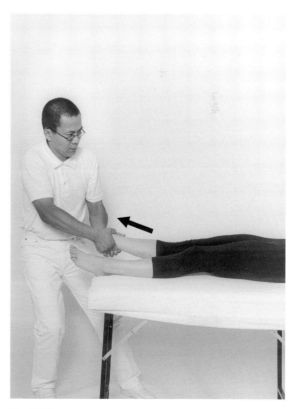

Fig. 2.29f

Upper Extremities

■ Shoulder

Symptoms of Vacuity

Slowly increasing pain, chronic pain, feeling of fatigue in the shoulder region, pale tongue with white fur, fine pulse.

Symptoms of Repletion

Suddenly occurring pain, pain that is more severe at night than during the day, localized sensitivity to cold, tongue with white fur, superficially stringlike pulse.

Shoulder Syndrome

Pain that can be associated with the shoulder as a functional unit.

For Symptoms of Vacuity

An 按 **Pressing**

- With the thumb
- On the seated patient
- ST-36
- BL-23

For Symptoms of Repletion

An 按 **Pressing**

- CV-4
- BL-18

General Treatment

An 按 **Pressing**

- On the seated patient
- Treatments on the affected side of the shoulders
- GB-20
- The pushing direction of your thumb tip points medially and cranially in an imaginary line to the opposite eye.
- GB-21
- SI-14
- SI-11
- SI-10
- LI-14
- LI-11

Tui 推 **Pushing**

- With the ball of the hand
- On the seated patient
- On both sides on top of the bladder channel, from the cervicothoracic transition down to the sacrum
- Five to 10 times per side
→ **Fig. 2.30**

 Make sure that the ball of the hand is firmly positioned. You can increase the pressure by propping your elbow against your flank and iliac crest and by accompanying the hand's downward stroke with a flexion in the knees and hip.

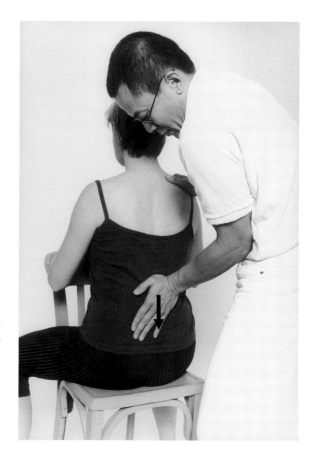

Fig. 2.30

Rou 揉 **Kneading**

- With the ball of the hand
- Above the trapezius region and paravertebral from the cervicothoracic transition to the lower cervical spine on the side of the affected shoulder. You can also treat the same area with *gun* by means of the ulnar edge of the hand.
- Three to 5 minutes
→ **Fig. 2.31**

Gun 滚 **Rolling**

- With the ulnar edge of the hand
- On the seated patient, with the arm raised to the side (up to 70°)
- Standing next to and facing the patient, place the foot that is closer to the patient on the sitting surface and support the patient's arm with your thigh. The arm should be kept in approximately 30° forward flexion and approximately 70–80° lateral flexion.
- Treatment proceeds upward from the distal (humeral) attachment of the deltoid, continuing above the front, middle, and back sections of the deltoid. Perform 30–40 rolling movements in each section.
→ **Fig. 2.32**

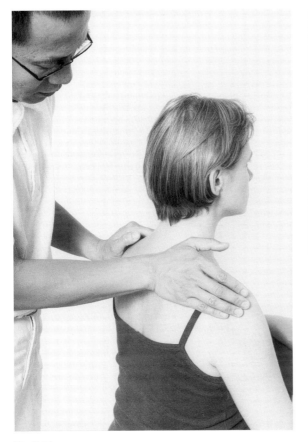

Fig. 2.31

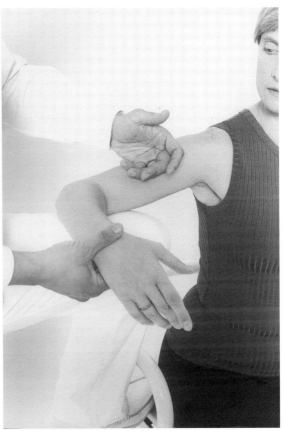

Fig. 2.32

Dui An 对按 **Grasping and Kneading**

- On the seated patient with the arm lifted to the side (position as in the *gun* technique, see above)
- With the index finger and thumb (in pinch grip), grip the deltoid muscle from craniolateral at SI-10 and LU-2 and apply small kneading movements.
- About five to 10 times
→ **Fig. 2.33a, b**

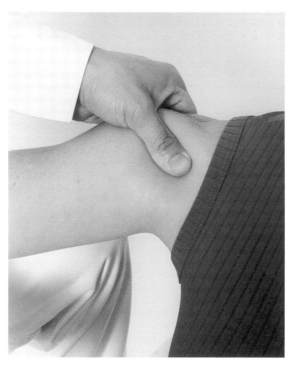

Fig. 2.33a

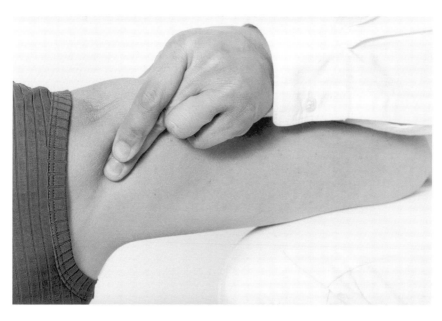

Fig. 2.33b

Zhang Dui An 掌对法 **Pressing**

- On the seated patient with the arm lifted to the side (position as in the *gun* technique, see above)
- Clasp the shoulder from ventral and dorsal between the ball of the hand and the interlaced fingers, slowly push the resulting bulge of tissue (skin, deltoid) cranially, hold for 1–2 seconds, and release the pressure without losing skin contact.
- Three to five times

→ **Fig. 2.34**

Fig. 2.34

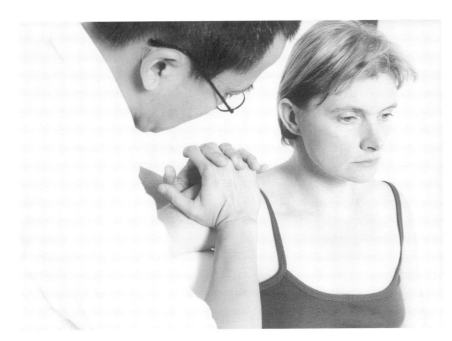

■ Specific Indications in the Shoulder

Impingement Syndrome

An 按 **Pressing**

- On the seated patient
- Hold the shoulder passively, as far as tolerated by the patient, in slight abduction and inward rotation. Now press in with the tip of the thumb on the greater tubercle (of the humerus), slowly proceeding from ventral to dorsal, three to five times, taking the severity of the patient's symptoms into consideration.
- On each point, maintain pressure for 5 seconds and then slowly release.
→ **Fig. 2.35**

An 按 **Pressing**

- With the tip of the thumb
- LU-2, on top

- Maintain pressure for up to 5 seconds and slowly release.
- One to two times

An Ban Fa 按扳法 **Pressing and Twisting**

Articular Capsule, Triceps Brachii
- On the seated patient, with the shoulder (humeroscapular joint) in anteversion and abduction of around 120° and maximum flexion in the elbow joint
- The practitioner stands to the side and back of the patient. The hand closer to the patient offers resistance on the top of the patient's shoulder and prevents the shoulder blade from moving along. Placed flat against the distal back side of the upper arm, the other hand supports and forces the shoulder into abduction, slowly building tension and slowly releasing.
- Five to eight times
→ **Fig. 2.36**

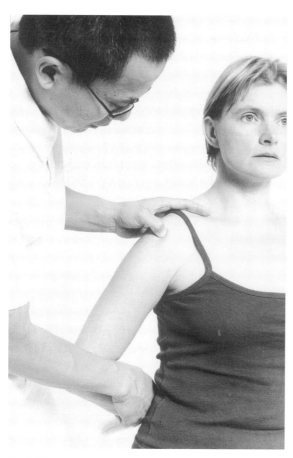

Fig. 2.35

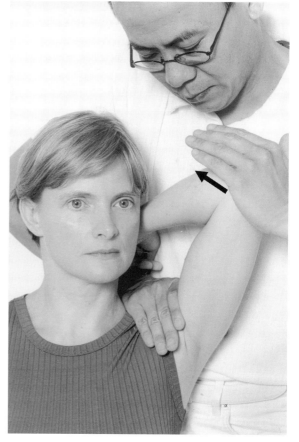

Fig. 2.36

Qian La Fa 牵拉法 **Traction and Pulling**

Dorsal Articular Capsule, Dorsal Deltoid, Infraspinatus
- On the seated patient
- Adduction of about 30° in the shoulder (humeroscapular joint) in front of the trunk, with 90° flexion in the elbow joint. The practitioner stands to the side and behind the patient.
- The hand on the treatment side applies a lateral push to the acromion and a forward rotation of the shoulder blade. Placed flat against the distal back side of the upper arm, the other hand supports and forces the shoulder into adduction, slowly building tension and slowly releasing.
- Five to eight times
→ **Fig. 2.37**

Qian Yin 牵引 **Traction**

- Grasp the patient's hand, abduct the affected shoulder 70–90°, and use the outside and back side of your distal upper arm to apply pressure to the inside of the patient's forearm, from a slight initial tension.
- Three to five times
→ **Fig. 2.38**

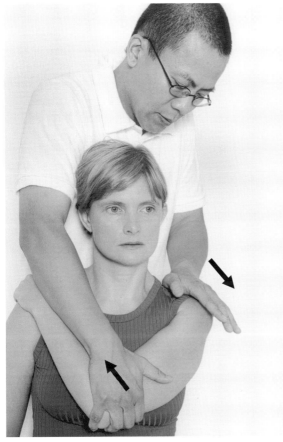

Fig. 2.37

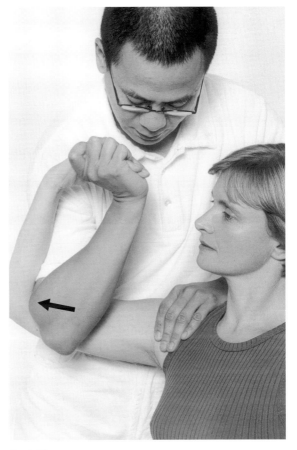

Fig. 2.38

Qian Yin 牵引 Traction

- On the seated patient with the arm raised 45° forward and 45° to the side
- Clasp the patient's metacarpus and carpus in both hands. The patient's trunk, which is supported from behind by the chair, serves as the "counterfort".

- Hold the pull for about 10–15 seconds.
- Five to eight times
→ **Fig. 2.39**

 You can also apply traction by clasping the ring and little finger with both of your corresponding fingers.

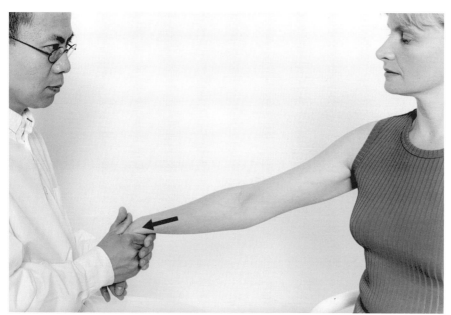

Fig. 2.39

Qian Yin 牵引 **Traction with Swinging Technique**

- Position yourself to the side and slightly in front of the patient and immobilize the top of the shoulder joint with the hand that is not actively manipulating. Clasp the patient's metacarpus and carpus and perform a quick jerky pull by means of a small inward rotation and swinging motion through the forearm.
- Five to eight times
→ **Fig. 2.40a, b**

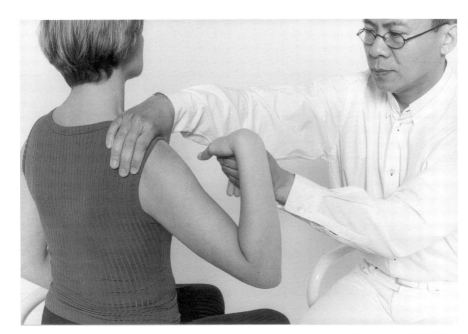

Fig. 2.40a

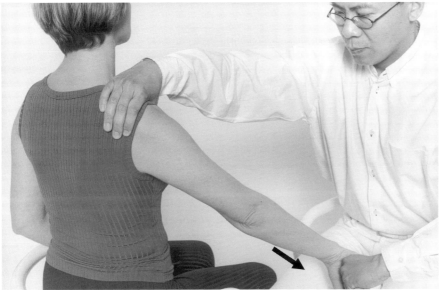

Fig. 2.40b

Frozen Shoulder (Adhesive Capsulitis)

Xuan Zhuan Fa   旋转法   **Rotating Mobilization**

- Stand to the side and in back of the patient. Cross your hands on the top of the patient's shoulder joint. The patient's flexed elbow joint lies in the crook of your arm.
- By bending the knees and hips rhythmically, you cause inward and outward circling movements in maximum abduction of 60–80°.
- Keep your shoulder area steady. Avoid swinging motions out of the shoulder. Rotate five to eight times clockwise and counterclockwise.

→ **Fig. 2.41a–c**

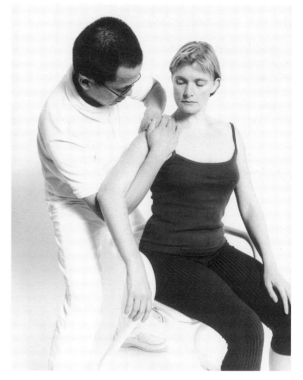

Fig. 2.41a

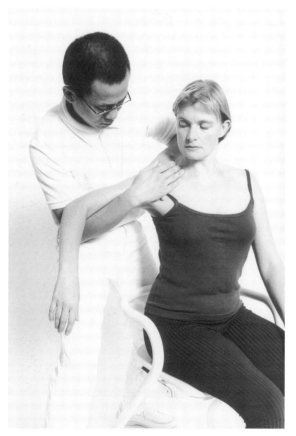

Fig. 2.41b

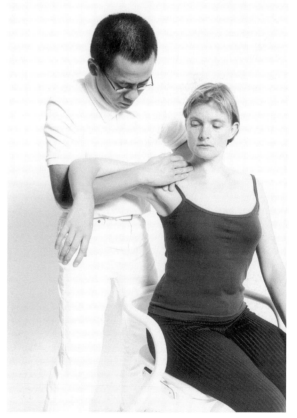

Fig. 2.41c

Qian Yin Dou Fa 牵引抖法 **Traction with Shaking**

- On the seated patient
- Traction with shaking movements, arm in 45° forward and 45° lateral flexion
- With interlaced fingers, clasp the patient's carpus and metacarpus with both hands. Perform shaking movements under traction. You create something like a standing wave with the intersection in the hand and shoulder joint.
- The treatment lasts about 10 seconds, five to eight times.

→ See **Fig. 2.39**

■ Elbow, Forearm, Hand

Humeroradial and Ulnar Epicondylitis

Musculotendinosis of the Flexors and Extensors of the Forearm

> ❗ We recommend a combined treatment of the medial and lateral side. Additional advice is found in Chapter 3 on "Treatment of Chronic Pain after Sport Injuries, Prevention" (pp. 82 ff)

An 按 **Pressing**

- With the thumb
- SI-14
- GB-20
- GB-21
- SI-10
- LI-14

Tui 推 **Pushing**

- With the ball of the hand
- On the seated patient
- On top of the bladder channel from the lower section of the cervical spine to the sacrum, on both sides
- Three to five times

→ **Fig. 2.42**

Gun 滚 **Rolling**

- With the ulnar edge of the hand
- On the seated patient

→ **Fig. 2.43**

or

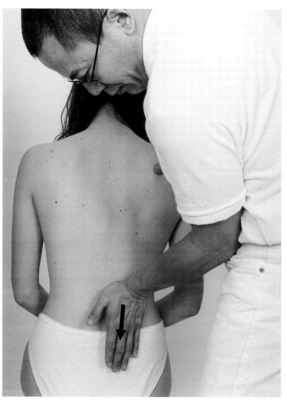

Fig. 2.42

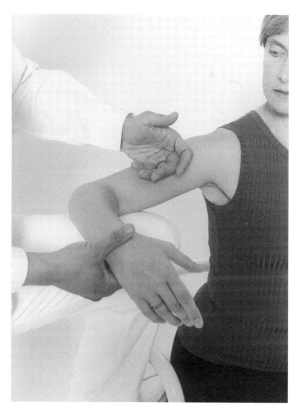

Fig. 2.43

Rou 揉 Kneading

- With the ball of the hand
- Starting in the area of the trapezius on the affected side and on top of the deltoid, 1 minute each
→ See **Fig. 2.4**

Gun 滚 Rolling

- With the ulnar edge of the hand
- On the seated patient
- Descending on top of the three *yang* channels of the arm from the distal forearm to the shoulder on the affected side, three to five times
→ See **Fig. 2.5**

Gun 滚 Rolling

- With the ulnar edge of the hand

or

Rou 揉 Kneading

- With the thumb
- LI-11, 3–5 minutes (**Fig. 2.44**)
- SI-8, 3–5 minutes
- HT-3, 3–5 minutes

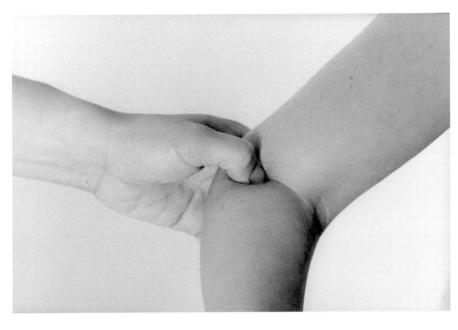

Fig. 2.44

Arthritis of the Hand and Finger Joints

Rou 揉 Kneading

- With the thumb
- On the muscle belly of the radial extensor
- Roughly between LI-8 and LI-10. We recommend also treating the ulnar extensors, in the area of SI-7 and SI-8.
- For 5–10 minutes

Qū Shen Fa 曲伸法 Flexion and Extension

- Patient and practitioner sit diagonally opposite each other. The outsides of the knees touch. Now grasp the patient's dorsal elbow region (e.g., on the right) with the thumb, index, and middle finger of your left hand. With the thumb, index, and middle finger of your right hand, clasp the patient's wrist.
- In a stretching motion, now bring the elbow joint close to the neutral position up to about 10° (avoid over-stretching). With the elbow joint in extension, perform a forced flexion on the patient's wrist joint and supinate the forearm, whereby the fingers extend passively.
- From this position, bring the elbow joint into a flexion that is approximately 10° from maximal flexion, stretch the wrist into maximum extension, and bring the forearm into pronation (inward rotation). The fingers of the patient's hand hereby move passively into functional position. Perform this combination of movements in an approximately 2-second rhythm 10 to 15 times.

→ **Fig. 2.45a, b**

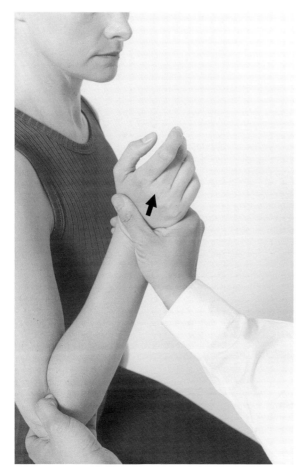

Fig. 2.45a

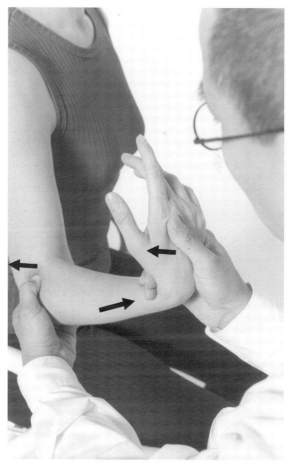

Fig. 2.45b

Qian Yin 牵引 **Traction with Mobilization of the Wrist**

- On the patient sitting upright and leaning against a backrest
- Raise the arm of the affected side in the shoulder approximately 50–60° forward and 45° to the side. The forearm is in pronation (inward rotation), the elbow is extended.
- Clasp the patient's metacarpus and carpus with both of your hands. In rhythmic alternations, move the wrist slowly and with gentle pulls into extension and flexion as well as ulnarly and radially, each to the maximum position.
- Three to five passes
→ **Fig. 2.46**

 It is essential that the patient's shoulders and upper arms are on the whole relaxed. The only counterpoint to the traction is provided by the weight of the patient's upper body, leaning back slightly against the backrest.

Qian Yin 牵引 **Traction**

- On the seated patient
- On the five fingers of the side affected by radiating pain
- The arm is extended in the elbow and wrist joint, raised about 45° to the front and side. With one hand, immobilize the distal forearm. With the three ulnar fingers of the other hand, clasp one finger and gradually build the pull through the finger, metacarpus, and wrist, hold for 2–3 seconds, and release.
- Once per finger
→ See **Fig. 2.12a, b**

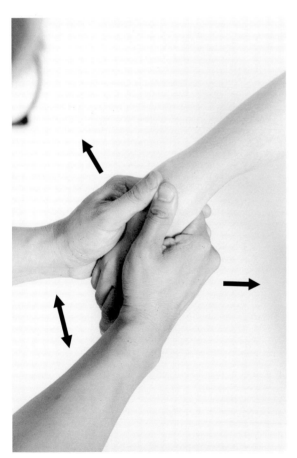

Fig. 2.46

Lower Extremities

■ Hip Joint

Coxalgia, Coxarthrosis

General Treatment

An 按 **Pressing**

- With the elbow
- In lateral position
- GB-29 (**Fig. 2.47**)
- In prone position
- GB-30

An 按 **Pressing**

- With the thumb
- In prone position
- GB-31
- GB-34
- BL-34
- BL-40
- BL-57

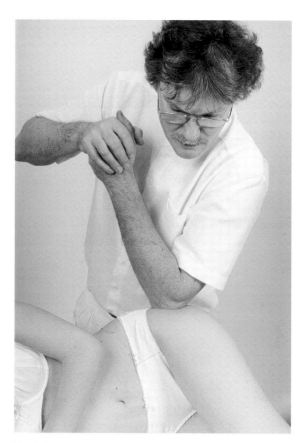

Fig. 2.47

An 按 **Pressing**

- With the elbow or in pinch grip with both thumbs and index fingers
- In prone position

- In the lumbar area on both sides on the eye points of the back against the tip of the transverse process of L3 → **Figs. 2.48** and **2.49**

→ Compare the section on the "Spinal Column" (pp. 19 ff).

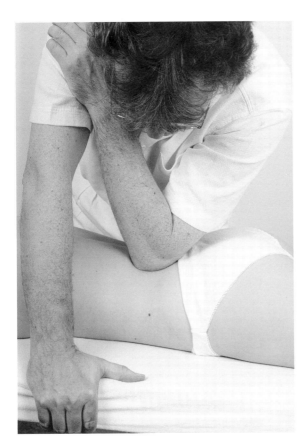

Fig. 2.48

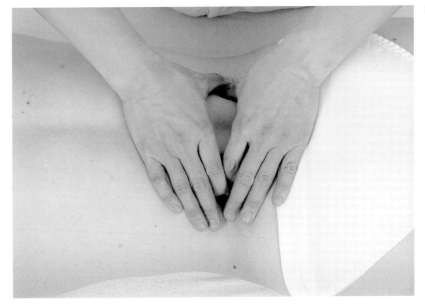

Fig. 2.49

Tui 推 **Pushing**

- With the ball of the hand
- In prone position
- Treat the bladder channel on both sides, descending from the cervical spine to the foot.
- Three to five times

→ See **Fig. 2.19a–d**

Tui 推 **Pushing**

- With the ball of the hand
- In lateral position with the leg bent
- Treat the gallbladder channel on both sides, descending from the area of the trochanter down to the distal lower leg.
- Five to 10 times

→ **Fig. 2.50a, b**

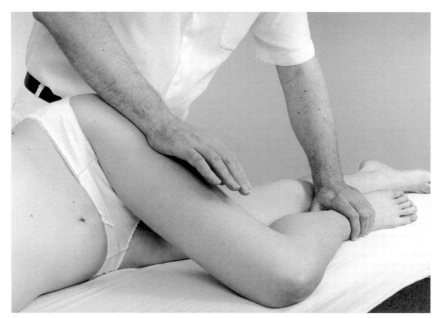

Fig. 2.50a

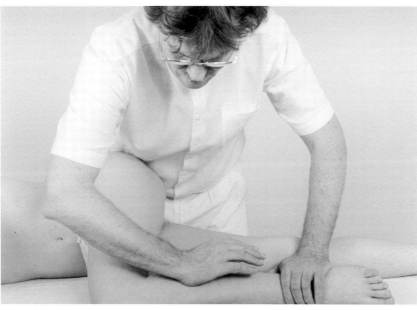

Fig. 2.50b

An Xi Ti Tun Fa 按膝提臀法 **Knee–Buttocks Counterpressure and Circular Movement**

Primarily Rotating Mobilization of the Lumbar Spine and Stretch of the Gluteal Muscles

- In supine position with the arms placed laterally on the table and the knees and hip in maximum flexion
- With your hand and forearm, immobilize the front sides of the upward-pointing ridges of the shinbones. Your other arm and forearm immobilize the buttocks in a wide embrace. Fixate (lock) your forearms against the trunk.
- The movement is caused by the practitioner by moving the legs and pelvis. The resulting circling move- ment on the patient points with the apex toward the area of the central and lower lumbar spine, toward the right and left.
- About 1 minute

→ **Fig. 2.51**

 As a general rule, generate only small circling movements.

- To further emphasize the stretch on the gluteus minimus, you can subsequently exert a straight push, without circling movement, with your forearm onto the upper end of the shinbone, while pulling up the other forearm that is immobilizing the patient's buttocks.

Fig. 2.51

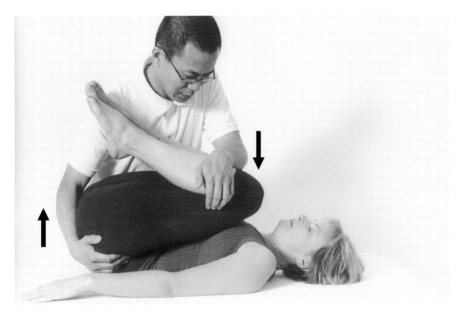

按膝提臀法

Kua Xuan Zhuan　旋转法　**Rotating Mobilization of the Hip Joint**

Outward and Inward Rotations in the Flexed Hip Joint
- In supine position
- Position yourself to the side by the lower end of the table. With the hand that is closer to the patient, clasp the distal lower leg and upper ankle; place the other hand ventrally on the knee.
- Treat clockwise and counterclockwise with alternating stretching and bending, abduction and adduction, up to five times in each direction.

→ **Fig. 2.52a, b**

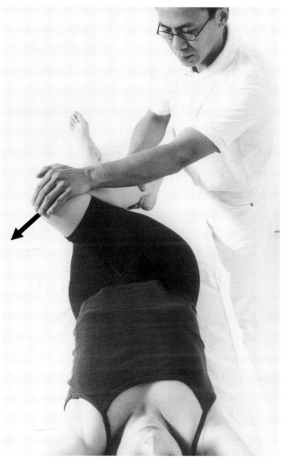

Fig. 2.52a

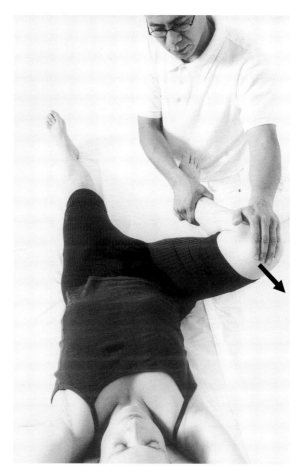

Fig. 2.52b

Qian Yin 牵引   **Traction**

Mild Traction of the Quadriceps Femoris and the Hip Joint

- In supine position with approximately 50° flexion in the hip and 100–110° flexion in the knee, the patient's foot placed on the table

- Sit on the table and immobilize the patient's forefoot under your thigh. Interlock your hands and clasp the distal section of the thigh from ventral.
- With a firm grip, pull the soft tissue slowly toward the knee, hold the pull for 3–5 seconds, and release.
- Five to 10 times

→ **Fig. 2.53**

Fig. 2.53

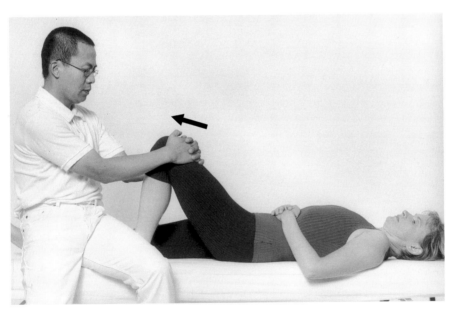

Si Zi 四字 **Numeral Four**

Stretch of the Ventral Hip Joint Capsule and Adductor Muscles
- In supine position
- Flex the hip joint to 90° and rotate outward and abduct as far as possible. Bend the knee over 90° and place the lower leg on top of the knee or thigh of the opposite side (numeral four).
- With one hand immobilize the crossways-lying lower leg. With the other carefully increase the abduction and outward rotation in the hip by pressing down on the medial side of the knee joint or thigh.
- Slowly build the tension, hold in maximum position for 5–10 seconds, and release.
- One to two times
→ **Fig. 2.54**

Qian Yin 牵引 **Traction of the Leg**

- In supine position
- Above the heel, grip the Achilles tendon and the region above the ankle. The thumb lies flat along the fibula or tibia (do not pinch). The second hand lies on the dorsum of the foot.
- Apply traction to the extended leg with 20° abduction and 30° flexion in the hip. Slowly build up the traction, hold 3–4 seconds, and release; approximately three to five tractions.
→ **Fig. 2.55**

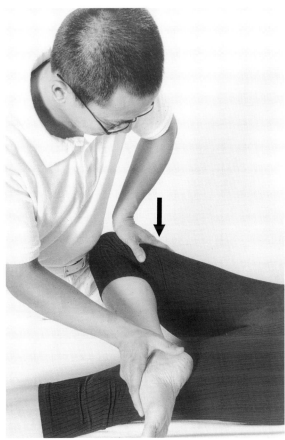

Fig. 2.54

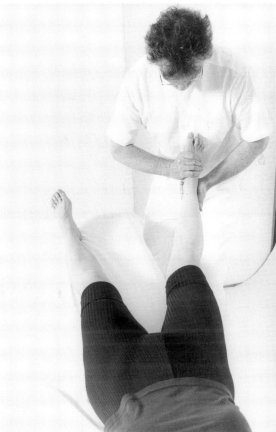

Fig. 2.55

An Ban Fa 按扳法 **Pressing and Twisting, Forced Hip Extension**

- In prone position
- Like the mobilizing treatment for the sacrum. The fixed resistance is not given in the sacrum but in the arch in the buttocks.
- With circling movements, on the right counterclockwise, on the left clockwise, three to five times
→ **Fig. 2.56**

> **!** Subsequently, you can hold the hip extension with pulling impulse in maximum adduction for approximately 3–5 seconds. Compare *an ban fa* in the section on the "Spinal Column" above (p. 19).

Tui 推 **Pushing**

- With the ball of the hand
- In lateral position
- On top of the gallbladder channel from the buttocks to the dorsum of the foot
- The patient's leg on the treatment side is flexed.
- Five to 10 times
→ See **Fig. 2.50a, b**

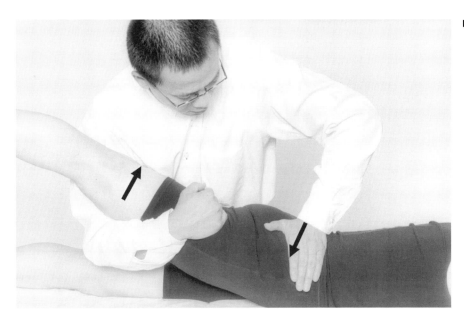

Fig. 2.56

Tui 推 **Pushing**

- With the ball of the hand
- In supine position
- On the stomach channel down from the hip area to the dorsum of the foot
- Three to five times
→ **Fig. 2.57**

Gun 滚 **Rolling**

- With the ulnar edge of the hand
- In lateral position
- With the patient's leg on the treatment side flexed, apply this technique to a roughly palm-sized area on top of the bulge of the greater trochanter; up to 3 minutes.
→ **Fig. 2.58**

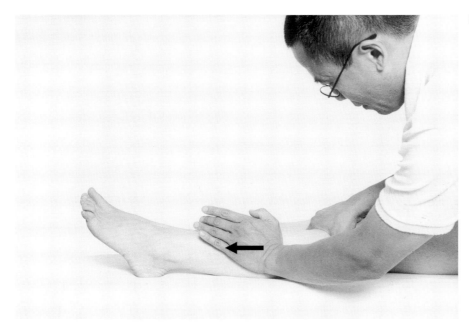

Fig. 2.57

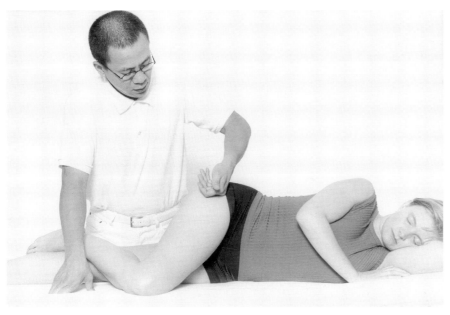

Fig. 2.58

Qian Yin 牵引 | Traction of the Ankle

- In supine position
- Stand at the foot of the table, facing the patient. With the right hand, clasp the Achilles tendon and heel from dorsal and pull. The leg is flexed approximately 30° in the hip or, in other words, lifted above the table 30°. With your left hand, grip the mid-foot and the area of the toes from medial so that the base joint of the large toe ends up lying in the crease of the base joints of your fingers. Now provide firm resistance from plantar with the thumb and ball of the thumb against the ball of the large toe and the large toe.
- From the practitioner's perspective, describe small circling movements in counterclockwise direction, whereby the upward movement results in greater traction when the forefoot is lifted, while the downward movement results in a greater pull on the forefoot when it is lowered.
- Five to eight circling movements, on both sides
→ **Fig. 2.59a, b**

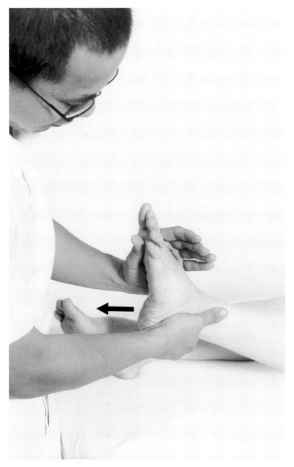

Fig. 2.59a

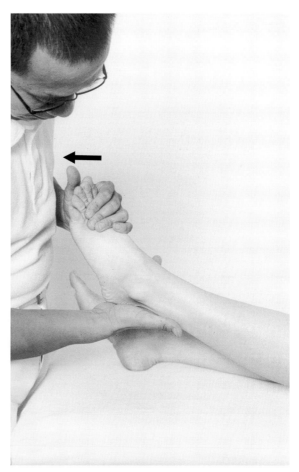

Fig. 2.59b

Qian Yin 牽引 **Traction of the Toes**

- In supine position
- Grip the toes on one or both sides, beginning with the little toe, one after the other from dorsal and plantar between thumb and index finger and pull with moderate force into functional position.
- With one hand, secure the foot in slight plantar flexion from dorsal at the heel and ankle so that the ankle is not pulled into extension during the traction.
- Once each
- → **Fig. 2.60**

■ Knee Joint

Gonalgia, Pain in the Capsule and Ligaments, Patellar Chondropathy

Pain that can be associated with the knee as a functional unit

General Treatment

An 按 **Pressing**

- With the tip of the elbow
- BL-29
- Eye points of the back (**Fig. 2.61**)
- With the thumb
- BL-54, BL-57

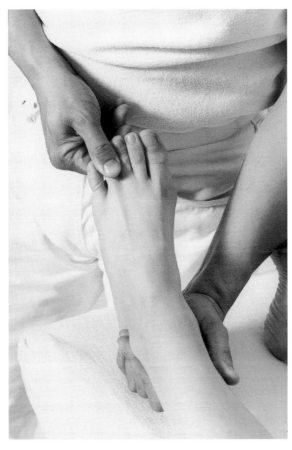

Fig. 2.60

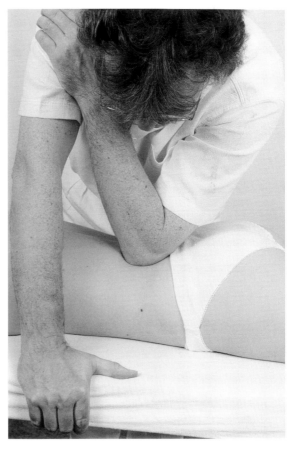

Fig. 2.61

Tui 推 **Pushing**

- With the ball of the hand
- In prone position
- On top of the bladder channel on both sides, descending from the cervical spine to the foot
- Five to 10 times

→ See **Fig. 2.19a–d**

Tui 推 **Pushing**

- With the ball of the hand
- In supine position
- Stomach, gallbladder (**Fig. 2.62**) and spleen channel caudally
- Three to five times

An 按 **Pressing**

- With the thumb
- GB-31, GB-34
- On the affected side
- Also ST-36
- SP-10, SP-9, SP-6

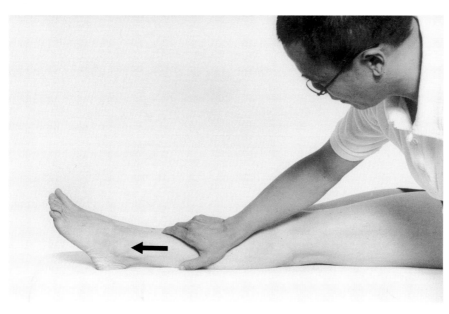

Fig. 2.62

Xuan Zhuan   旋转法   **Traction and Rotating Mobilization, Near the Knee**

- In half-lying position with the upper body comfortably propped up halfway and the legs extended. Clasp the patient's ankle area with your armpit, lateral chest wall, and upper arm. Grip the tibial plateau with both hands.

- Perform a traction with the knee joint in slight flexion of 10–30°. Under traction, apply varizing and valgizing movements to the knee joint so that the knee describes a continuous figure of eight.
- Up to three times
→ **Fig. 2.63a, b**

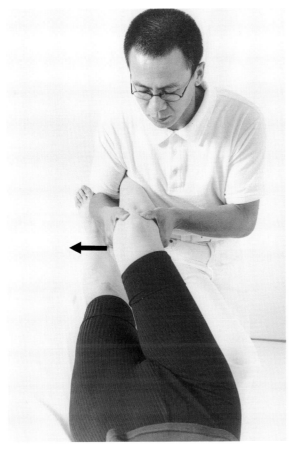

Fig. 2.63a

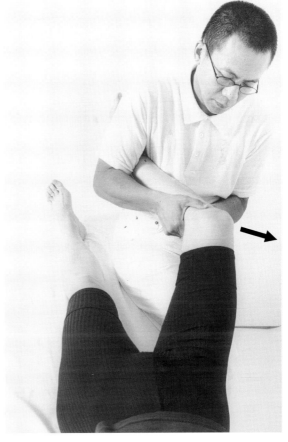

Fig. 2.63b

Patellar Chondropathy, Retropatellar Arthritis

Specific Treatment

Na Bin 拿髕 **Patellar Mobilization**

- In supine position, with the knee slightly flexed
- Place the five fingers of your hand in slightly opposing position with the tips pointing inward. Hereby, a crown-shaped finger position is created.
- Carefully grip the edge of the kneecap. Briefly lift the kneecap, then release it. The gripping and releasing is done rhythmically, slowly approximately 10–20 times.
→ **Fig. 2.64**

> **!** In patients with more severe synovial irritation and sensitivity to pressure at the edge of the joint surface and the periosteum, apply this gripping technique only with care and vary the placement of the finger tips.

Gonarthritis, Chondropathy, Chronic Global Knee Pain

An 按 **Pressing**

- Pressing on the eye points of the knee joint. These are two points on the lower edge of the patella, to both sides of the patella tendon. The exterior point lies slightly lateral to ST-35; the pressure direction is medially and laterally on both sides with the thumb, approximately to the center of Hoffa's fat pad.
- Treat the point slowly and rhythmically, several times, with gentle pressure.
- Carry out approximately three to five pushes with both thumb tips at the same time.
→ **Fig. 2.65**

> **!** Circling movements are expressly contraindicated here.

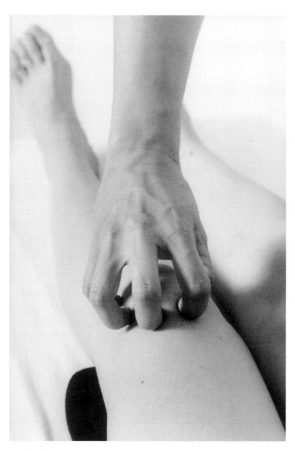

Fig. 2.64

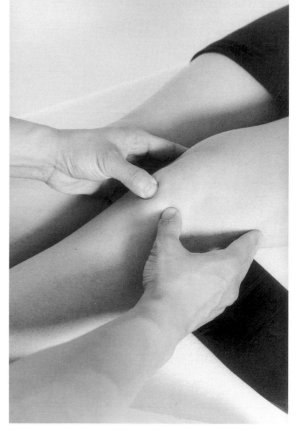

Fig. 2.65

Active Gonarthritis, Reduction of Swelling

Gun 滚 **Rolling**

- With the ulnar edge of the hand
- Rest the knee in slight flexion. The patient's upper body is positioned comfortably in slightly elevated supine position.

- Along the anterior upper recess of the knee joint, perform continuously rolling movements, advancing slowly from lateral to medial and back; 15–20 minutes.
→ **Fig. 2.66**

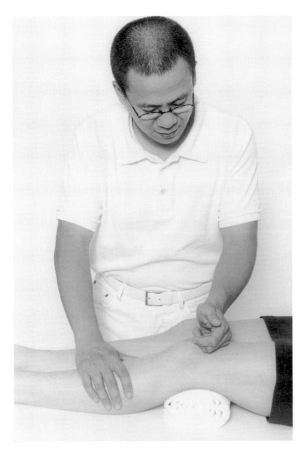

Fig. 2.66

Patellar Apex Syndrome, Jumper's Knee

An 按 **Pressing**

- With the tip of the thumb
- Beginning cranially against the attachment across the entire width of the patellar tendon, lateral or medial. At the patellar apex, perform small pushes with a short path and strong pressure, one each per new position against the bony layer below the tendon. You can apply pressure to between five and 10 pressure points across the entire width of the kneecap.
- Treat the pressure points in an orderly direction, that is, from lateral to medial or the other way around, only once each. Hereby, it is of utmost importance that the kneecap does not perform any evasive movements. You must therefore immobilize the upper edge of the kneecap with the other hand on the femoral condyle. The easiest way to do this is to secure the upper edge with the thumb.
- The treatment goal is to create a stimulation at the tendon attachment (microtrauma) with the tip of the thumb.
- Up to three passes

→ **Fig. 2.67**

→ Stretching techniques for the ischiocrural muscles are described on p. 43 (**Fig. 2.28**a) and p. 90.

Fig. 2.67

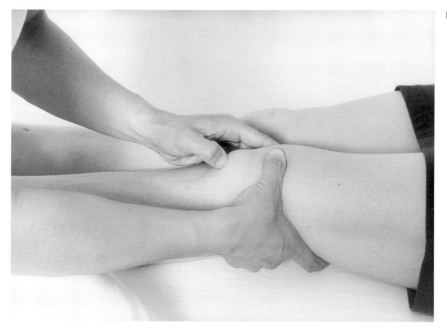

Irritable Knee, Chronic Synovitis

An 按 **Pressing**

- Sitting position or half-reclining
- Rub ST-34 against SP-10 in a pinching grip against each other with circling pressure movements deep down.
- Regulate the pressure carefully because both of these points tend to be very sensitive.
- Three to 5 minutes
- → **Fig. 2.68**

 Contraindicated in patients with gouty arthropathy. See general contraindications in Chapter 1 (p. 6).

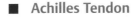 **Achilles Tendon**

Achillodynia, Tendomuscular Symptoms in the Soleus, Gastrocnemius, and Flexor Muscles of the Toes

Example of treatment on the left side. Position yourself on the left side of the table, facing the head, and place your right leg flexed on the table. Prop the patient's lower leg, with the knee slightly bent, against your thigh.

In this position perform the following:

Rou 揉 **Kneading**

- With the thumb
- BL-57
- → **Fig. 2.69**

And subsequently:
- With both thumbs
- On the Achilles tendon and calf in ascending direction
- Three to five times

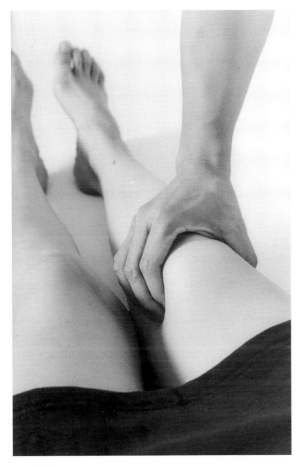

Fig. 2.68

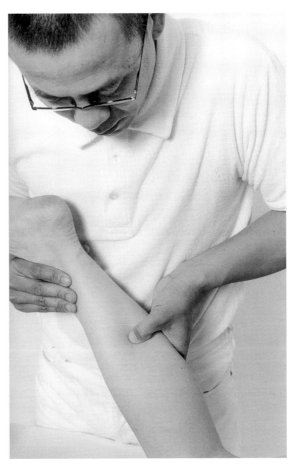

Fig. 2.69

Tui 推 **Pushing**

- With thumbs placed on top of each other
- Perform brief pushes of 1–2 cm each from the heel, on the Achilles tendon, and continuing proximally on the soleus and gastrocnemius.
- Three to five passes
→ **Fig. 2.70**

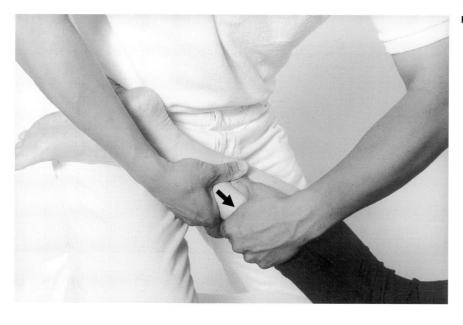

Fig. 2.70

Qian Yin 牵引 Traction

- In prone position
- Stand at the foot of the table. The knee is flexed approximately 30–40°. Take hold of the back of the forefoot and middle foot and interlock your thumbs across the distal sole of the foot. In this position, place the foot on your chest.
- Guide slow rhythmic movements by bending and stretching your hip and the knee and ankle joints.
- Three to five times with a careful stretch in the calf muscles.
→ **Fig. 2.71**

Ti Dou 提抖 Traction and Shaking

- In prone position
- The knee is flexed 90°. Place your hand that is located closer to the head down flat from dorsal. Bring the ankle joint into a 20–30° flexion with the foot slightly tipped, providing support at the back of the foot with the hand that lies closer to the foot. Now perform shaking movements with the hand closer to the head via the heel, causing a rapidly changing rotation along the longitudinal axis of the lower leg.
- A slight plantar flexion in the foot is important to relax the dorsal lower leg muscles; approximately 30 seconds.
→ **Fig. 2.72**

➡ For additional information, see Chapter 3 on "Treatment of Chronic Pain after Sport Injuries, Prevention" (pp. 82 ff).

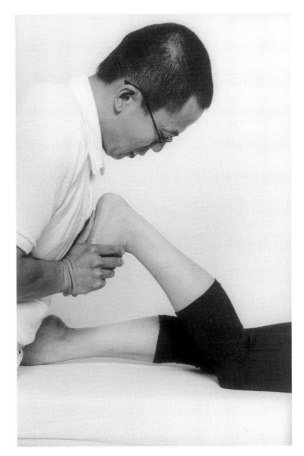

Fig. 2.71

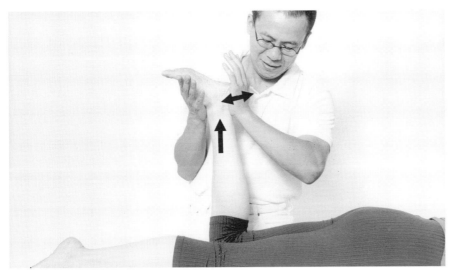

Fig. 2.72

■ Lower Leg and Foot

Tendomyotic Complaints in the Anterior and Posterior Lower Leg Muscles, the Ankle, and the Articular Connections of the Foot

General Treatment

An 按 Pressing

- With the thumb
- ST-41
- LR-4
- KI-6
- KI-3
- KI-1 (**Fig. 2.73**)
- GB-40
- BL-62

Metatarsalgia, Symptoms of Overstrain in the Transverse and Longitudinal Arches of the Foot

Mu Jian An 拇尖按 Pressing

- In supine position
- The knee on the treatment side is flexed 30–40°. Stand at the foot of the table.
- With the gripping surfaces of fingers 2 to 5, clasp the distal arch of the foot. With the distal phalanges of the thumbs lying next to each other, place the tips of the thumbs on the ball of the forefoot, beginning between the first and second metatarsal bones.
- Look for deep contact and treat the four spaces between the bones, one after the other, with slow ascending and descending rubbing movements, three to four times each per direction; up to three passes.

→ **Fig. 2.74**

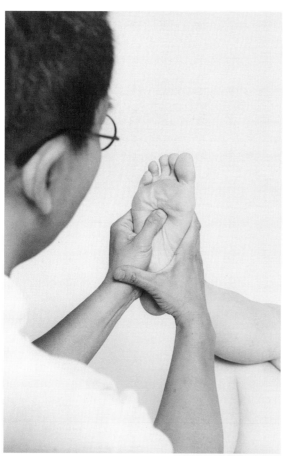

Fig. 2.73

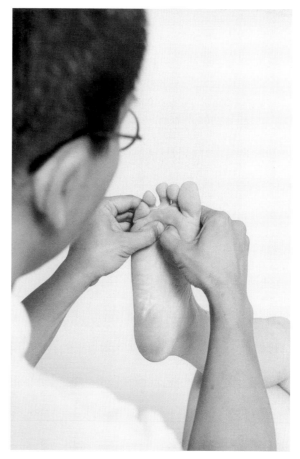

Fig. 2.74

Dui An 对按 **Grasping and Kneading**

- With interlocked fingers
- Grip the middle foot and forefoot from the dorsum of the foot. Interlock the thumbs on the sole without any great amount of pressure. Press the lateral and medial edges of the foot together in such a way that the transverse arch is increased.
- Slowly increase the pressure, hold for 3 seconds, and then release it, up to three times.
→ **Fig. 2.75**

Qian Yin 牵引 **Traction**

Calf Muscles, Plantar Fascia, and Transverse Arch of the Foot
- In prone position
- Grip the forefoot in such a way that you can also stretch the longitudinal arch. Secured in this way, place the forefoot in front of your chest. Slowly increase the pressure, hold for 3 seconds, and then release it.
- One to three times
→ Gripping position, see **Fig. 2.71**

Heel Spur and Pain in the Plantar Fascia

Tui 推 **Pushing**

- With the thumb
- In prone position
- The hand closer to the patient clasps the ankle, the thumb of the other hand pushes three paths in a row on the plantar fascia from the ball of the heel to the forefoot, applying strong pressure.
- Two to three passes
→ **Fig. 2.76**

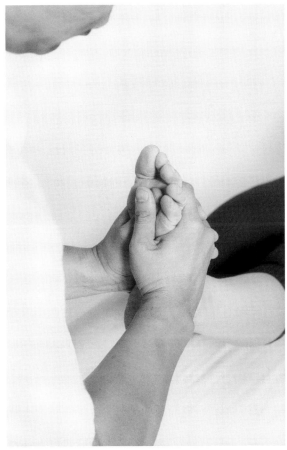

Fig. 2.75

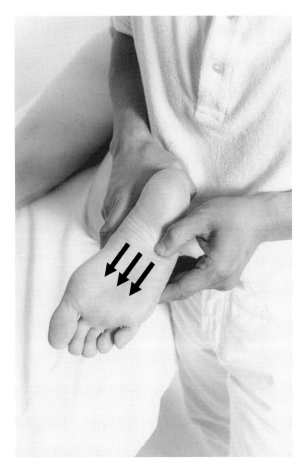

Fig. 2.76

Ji 挤 Tapping

- With the ulnar side of the closed fist
- In prone position, with the knee bent at a right angle. The other hand immobilizes the rear foot and ankle.
- Apply loose and slightly springing knocks.
- Five to 10 times
→ **Fig. 2.77**

An 按 Pressing

- With the tips of the thumbs
- In the prone position with the knee bent at a right angle
- The fingers provide resistance at the forefoot. Starting from the tip of the heel, apply pressure by progressing simultaneously across the lateral and medial edge of the ball, repositioning the thumbs in approximately 1-cm segments.
- Three to five passes
→ **Fig. 2.78**

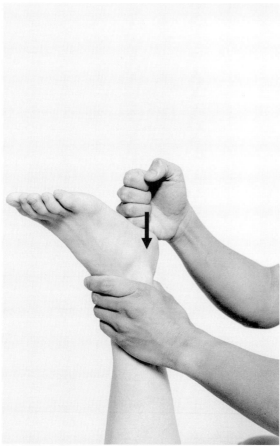

Fig. 2.77

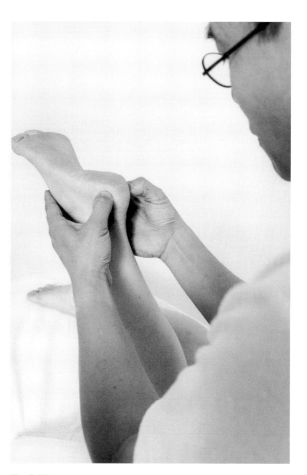

Fig. 2.78

Qian Yin 牽引 **Traction of the Toes**

- In supine position
- Grip the toes on one or both sides, beginning with the little toe, one after the other from dorsal and plantar between thumb and index finger and pull with moderate force into functional position.
- With one hand, secure the foot in slight plantar flexion from dorsal at the heel and ankle so that the ankle is not pulled into extension during the traction.
- Once each
→ **Fig. 2.79**

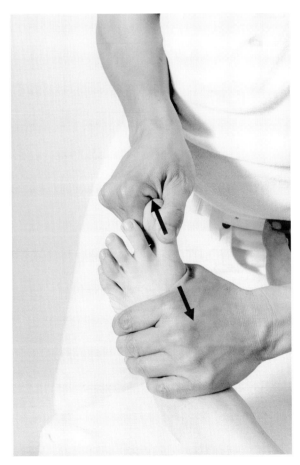

Fig. 2.79

3 Sports Indications: Treatment of Chronic Pain after Sport Injuries, Prevention

Chronified Shoulder Pain, Subacromial Bursitis, Tendinosis of the Long Biceps Tendon (e.g., in Throwers, Fencers, and Swimmers)

➡️ Pretreatments are found in the section on "Upper Extremities" in Chapter 2 (p. 46).

An Ban Fa 按扳法 **Pressing and Twisting**

- In the seated position with the shoulder in maximum elevation of 160–180° to the front and to the side, with the elbow flexed
→ **Fig. 3.1a**

- Grasp the back of the distal forearm and bring the shoulder joint into further abduction.
- Three to five times

❗ This treatment is also possible on a doorframe, for example. Here you have to make sure that the passive push on the back side of the distal forearm does not come from ventral but more from the lateroventral direction.

→ **Fig. 3.1b**

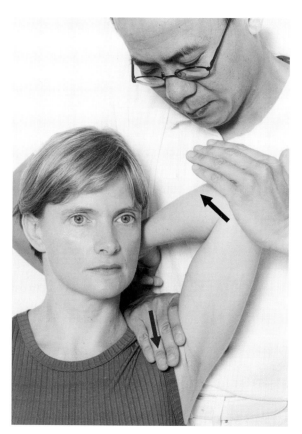

Fig. 3.1a

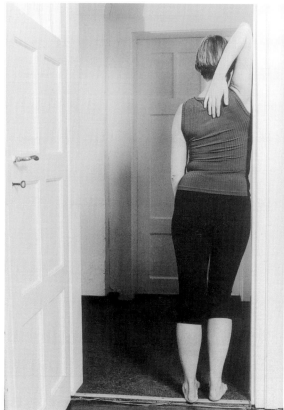

Fig. 3.1b

Qian La Fa 牵拉法 **Traction and Pulling**

- Self-treatment in the seated position
- Stretch of the dorsal shoulder muscles with the upper arm raised forward 70–80°, elbow flexed, and increased adduction, by placing the hand on the distal, dorsal upper arm
- Three to five times

→ **Fig. 3.2a, b**

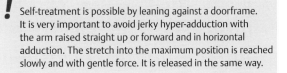 Self-treatment is possible by leaning against a doorframe. It is very important to avoid jerky hyper-adduction with the arm raised straight up or forward and in horizontal adduction. The stretch into the maximum position is reached slowly and with gentle force. It is released in the same way.

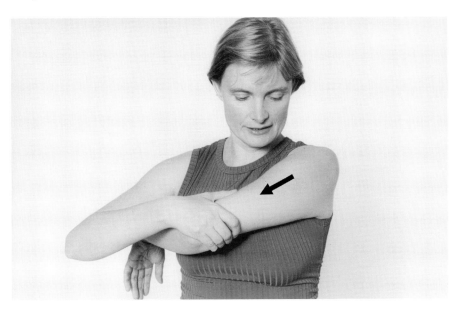

Fig. 3.2a

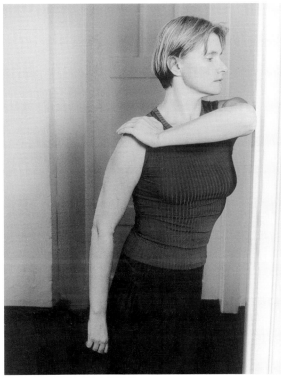

Fig. 3.2b

Sprain Injuries of the Finger Joints (e.g., Volleyball Injuries), Tendinosis of the Hand and Forearm

An 按 Pressing

- LI-11
- HT-3

Gun 滚 Rolling

- With the ulnar edge of the hand
- On the seated patient with slight elbow flexion and extended wrist. Treat from distal to proximal on the radial and ulnar flexors of the wrist, for about 2–3 minutes.
→ See **Fig. 2.5** in Chapter 2

Na 拿 Grasping

- With the patient's finger slightly extended or in functional position, work the radial and ulnar side of the finger in rapid succession from the base joint to the tip and back, using a pinch grip between the tips of your thumb and index finger.
- In the same way on the volar and dorsal side
- Two to three times
→ **Fig. 3.3**

Qian Yin Lü 牵引捋 Traction with Casting Off

- On the seated patient
- Clamp the patient's fingers, one after the other, gently between your index and middle finger and pull while loosening the grip in such a way that the patient's finger glides through.
- With the other hand, immobilize the wrist; three to five times per finger.
→ Gripping positions, see **Fig. 2.12a, b** in Chapter 2

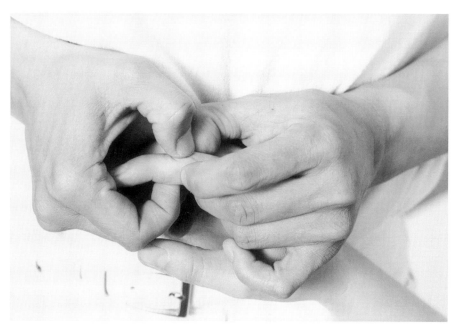

Fig. 3.3

Qian La Lü   牵拉捋   **Traction with Pulling on the Extensor Tendons of the Thumb**

- Immobilize the patient's thumb with your three fingers in the palm of your hand. Your thumb and index finger clasp the ball of the thumb. Apply a mild pull.
- With the tip of the thumb of your other hand, stroke deeply and slowly over the tendons and slide bearings of the extensor tendons distally to the saddle joint.
- Three to five times
→ **Fig. 3.4**

Qian Yin   牵引   **Traction with Mobilization of the Wrist**

- On the upright sitting patient, supported by a backrest
- Raise the arm of the affected side in the shoulder approximately 50–60° forward and abduct approxi-

mately 45°. The forearm is in pronation (inward rotation), the elbow is extended.
- Clasp the patient's metacarpus and carpus with both of your hands. In rhythmic alternations, move the wrist slowly and with gentle pulls into extension and flexion as well as ulnarly and radially, each to the maximum position.
- Three to five passes
→ **Fig. 3.5**

> **!** It is essential that the patient's shoulders and upper arms are mostly relaxed. The only counterpoint to the traction is provided by the weight of the patient's upper body, leaning back slightly against the backrest.

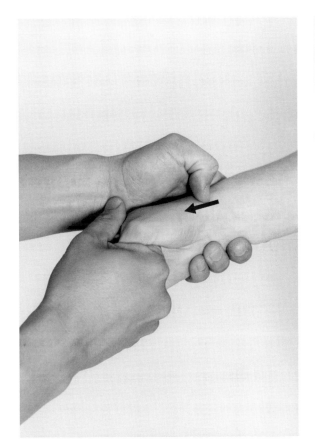

Fig. 3.4

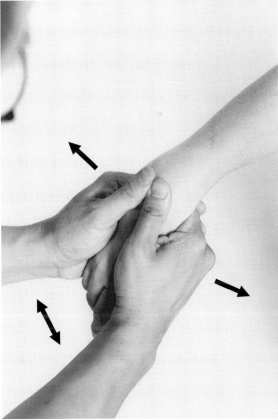

Fig. 3.5

Adductor Tendinopathy in the Thigh

Tui 推 **Pushing**

- In prone position
- Descending with the ball of the hand on both sides on top of the bladder channel, from the neck to the foot
- Three to five times

An 按 **Pressing**

- With the elbow
- BL-23
- GB-29 (**Fig. 3.6**)
- GB-30

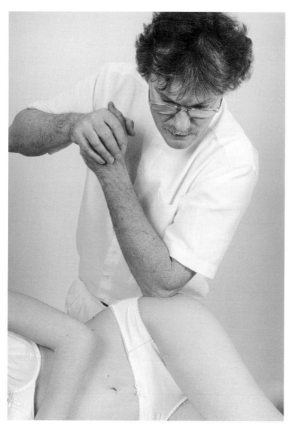

Fig. 3.6

An 按 **Pressing**

- In supine position
- With the thumbs on top of each other, supported by the fingers on the thigh
- Stand on the opposite side from the leg that you are treating. With strong, slowly increasing pressure on top of the adductors, ascending from distal to proximal, from the origin to the attachment, five to six times.
- Work this stretch five to six times in a row.

→ **Fig. 3.7**

Si Zi 四字 **Numeral Four**

With a Stretch of the Ventral Hip Joint Capsule and Adductor Muscles
- In supine position
- Flex the hip joint to 90° and rotate outward and abduct as far as possible. Bend the knee over 90° and place the lower leg on top of the knee or thigh of the opposite side (numeral four).
- With one hand, immobilize the transversely positioned lower leg; with the other, carefully apply pressure (downward) on the medial side of the knee joint or thigh to increase the abduction and outward rotation of the hip.
- Slowly build the tension, hold in maximum position for 3 seconds, and release.
- One or two times

→ See **Fig. 2.54** in Chapter 2

Tui 推 **Pushing**

- With the ball of the hand
- In prone position
- On the bladder channel from the neck to the foot
- Three to five times

An 按 **Pressing**

- With the elbow
- In lateral position
- On GB-29, building slowly and releasing
- One or two times

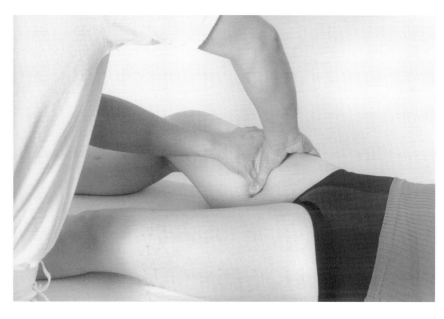

Fig. 3.7

Gun 滚 **Rolling**

- With the ulnar edge of the hand
- In lateral position with flexed hips and knee, on the greater trochanter, up to 5 minutes

Tui 推 **Pushing**

- With the ball of the hand
- In lateral position, descending on the gallbladder channel from the hip to the foot
- Five to 10 times
→ **Fig. 3.8a, b**

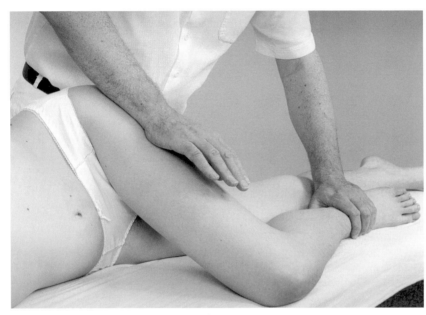

Fig. 3.8a

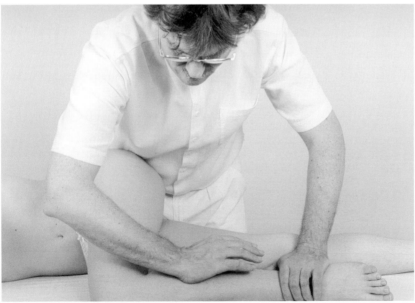

Fig. 3.8b

Pain in the Proximal Third of the Biceps Femoris and the Proximal Ischiocrural Muscles (e.g., in Sprinters and Middle Distance Runners)

Tui 推 Pushing

- In prone position
- On the bladder channel from the neck to the foot
- Three to five times

An 按 Pressing

- With the elbow
- On the eye points of the back (see the section on the "Spine" in Chapter 2, p. 30, **Fig. 2.16**)
- GB-29, GB-30

An 按 Pressing

- With the thumbs placed on top of each other or with the elbow
- In prone position
- On the biceps femoris descending from the tuberosity of the ischium on the back side of the thigh, from proximal to distal, approximately five to six times
- One or two times
- → **Fig. 3.9a, b**

> **!** This treatment can be very painful. Bracing yourself against the edge of the table helps in controlling the application of force and keeping your balance.

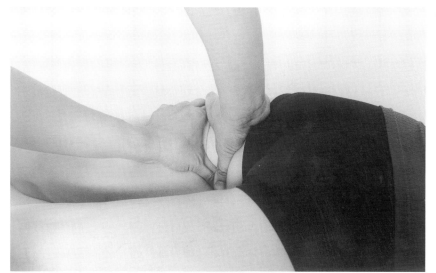

Fig. 3.9a

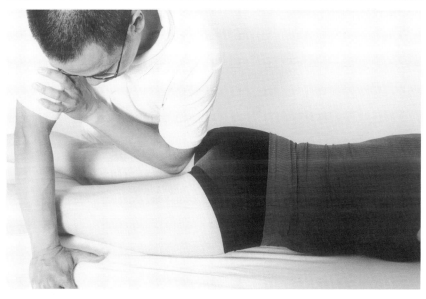

Fig. 3.9b

Qian Yin   牵引   **Traction of the Ischiocrural and Calf Muscles**

- Position yourself by the foot of the table, looking at the head of the table.
- With the patient in supine position, passively raise the patient's leg, extended in the knee, as far as possible, as if in a straight-leg-raising test. Place the calf in front of your shoulder. The hands with interlocked fingers offer resistance by the distal thigh. The patient's ankle joint initially remains extended. Keep your trunk upright.
- The increase and decrease in tension is caused by moving your trunk forward and backward, in a movement that arises exclusively from bending and stretching the hip, knee, and ankle joints.
- On both sides three to five times
- With sufficient tolerance, you can vary the method by slowly increasing tension with inward and outward rotations as well as by forcibly stretching the calf muscles via the ankle joint; up to three rotations per direction.

→ See **Fig. 2.28a–c** in Chapter 2

 Sensitivity to rotations in the ankle joint can create considerable limitations for this method.

Patellar Apex Syndrome, Patellar Chondropathy

Jing Dun   静蹲   **Isometric Strengthening**

- Self-treatment in the standing position
- Place the feet shoulder-width apart, parallel to each other, and with equal weight on the heel and forefoot. Bend the knees approximately 10°, straighten the pelvis, and slightly reduce the lordosis in the lumbar spine.
- Remain standing without shifting weight, until the muscles begin to shake slightly, then hold the tension for another 10–20 seconds, and finally release the legs.
- Perform this exercise twice a day.

→ **Fig. 3.10**

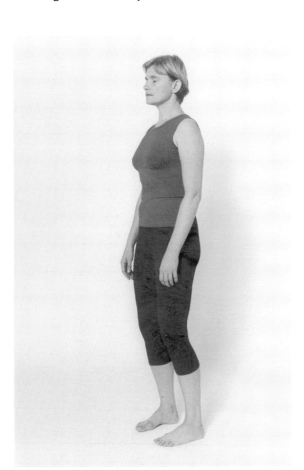

Fig. 3.10

Achillodynia

➡ Supplementary treatment techniques are found in the section on the "Lower Extremities" in Chapter 2 (pp. 59 ff, 77).

Qian Yin 牵引 **Traction**

- Self-treatment in the standing position
- Stretch one leg forward slightly. With the knees and hips slightly flexed, prop the toes and ball of the forefoot against a doorpost or the wall, placing the heel firmly on the ground. The dorsal flexion of the foot is increased by lightly flexing and advancing the knee joint (stretching the calf muscles).
- Build the tension slowly to the limit of tolerance, hold for 3–5 seconds, and release slowly, on both sides, three to five times.
- You should perform this exercise before and after a training session.
- → **Fig. 3.11**

Preparation for a Competition

By means of the following methods, it is possible to attain a calm mood on the day before the event. They can also be helpful in preparing for an examination. These techniques improve your ability to sleep through the night.

Tui 推 **Pushing**

- With the ball of the hand
- In prone position
- On the bladder channel from the top of the head to the upper cervical spine, separately on both sides three to five times, markedly slow pushing
- You can also treat both sides simultaneously.

Rou 揉 **Kneading**

- With the thumbs
- GB-20 (**Fig. 3.12**) and
- EX-5 (*an mian*)
- One or 2 minutes

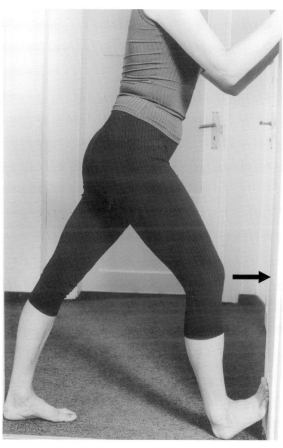

Fig. 3.11

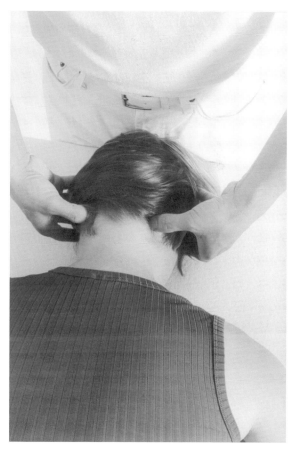

Fig. 3.12

Tui 推 Pushing

- With the ball of the hand
- In prone position
- On the bladder channel from the neck to the foot, markedly slow pushing. Treat the channels on both sides, one after the other.
- Three times

An 按 Pressing

- With the tip of the thumb
- In supine position
- On both sides of the bladder channel, beginning on the hairline at BL-4 upward to the vertex
- Subsequently using the same technique with one hand on the Governing Vessel upward from GV-24 to the vertex and back of the head
- Three to five times each

Fen Tui 分推 Lateral Pushing

- With the radial edge of the thumbs
- Stroke on the skin of the forehead parallel above the eyebrows to the EX-2 (*tai yang*).
- Three to five times
→ **Fig. 3.13**

Gua 刮 Scratching

- In supine position
- Bring the fingers 2 to 5 to the light functional position (flexion). Place the tips (with short nails) straight

down into the scalp and stroke the gallbladder channel and its vicinity in front of, above, and behind the ear.
- Three to five times
→ **Fig. 3.14**

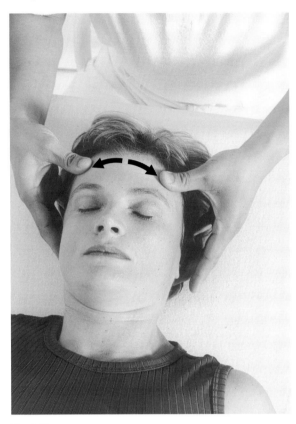

Fig. 3.13

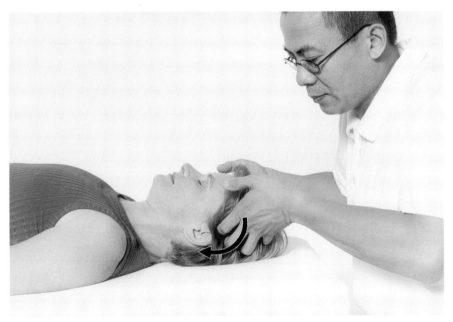

Fig. 3.14

An 按 **Pressing**

- In supine position
- It is important to execute this treatment slowly and calmly.
- Treat the two sides separately, first on the upper extremities, then on the lower extremities.
- LU-1
- ST-36
- SP-6
- GB-34
- GB-43
- LR-3

Yi Shou 意守 **Concentration and Relaxation**

- In supine position
- To conclude treatment, bring the body to a comfortable position. Sit down next to the table and place one hand without a lot of pressure on the middle of the abdomen at the level of the navel.
- The contestant/examinee should breathe slowly from the diaphragm and may also fall asleep, 15–20 minutes.
- → **Fig. 3.15**

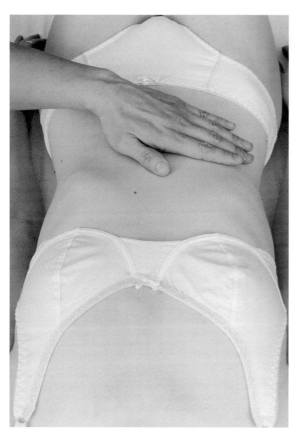

Fig. 3.15

4 Internal Medicine Indications: Psychovegetative Disorders, Headaches

Colds and Flus, Disorders of the Upper Respiratory Tracts

Leading Symptom: Sensation of Cold

Accompanied by shivering, headache, drowsiness, lack of thirst, no sweating.

Leading Symptom: Sensation of Heat

Accompanied by sweating, sore throat, headache, dry mouth.

For Sensation of Cold

An 按 **Pressing**

- BL-12
- LU-7

For Sensation of Heat

An 按 **Pressing**

- GV-14
- LI-4, on both sides (see Chapter 1, **Fig. 1.11**, p. 12)
- GB-20, on both sides

Chronic Bronchitis, Bronchial Asthma

Symptoms of Vacuity

Forceless cough, pale facial complexion, tendency to sweat even when resting, subjective cold sensation and sensitivity to cold, soft stools, dry mouth and throat, dark red tongue with no fur, moist hands and feet, deep and stringlike pulse.

Symptoms of Repletion

Forceful cough, loud breathing, impatient behavior, loud voice, distended abdomen, solid stools, combination of dry mouth and bitter taste, tongue with white fur, yellowish bronchial phlegm, stringlike and slippery pulse.

General Treatment

Tui 推 **Pushing**

- With the balls of both hands
- In prone position
- Stand at the head of the table and treat the bladder channel from C6 down to the sacrum, on both sides simultaneously.
- Apply three pushes in each expiratory phase.

→ See **Fig. 1.3** in Chapter 1

Tui 推 **Pushing**

- With thumbs placed on top of each other
- On the bladder channel one after the other (right/left) also caudally
- Here, it is sufficient to treat the area between the lower cervical spine and the middle thoracic spine, three times on each side.

→ **Fig. 4.1**

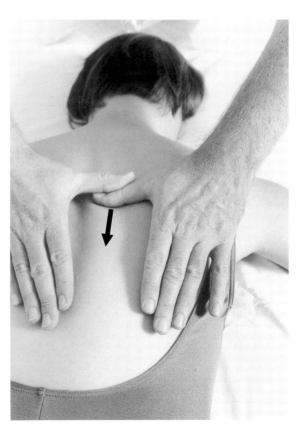

Fig. 4.1

Heng Ca 橫擦 **Transverse Scrubbing**

- With the flat palm of the hand
- In supine position
- On the chest in the area between the second and fourth rib rapidly 100–200 times
→ **Fig. 4.2**

Heng Ca 橫擦 **Transverse Scrubbing**

- With the flat palm of the hand
- In prone position
- On the upper back in the area between the seventh cervical and the third thoracic vertebra rapidly 100–200 times
→ **Fig. 4.3**

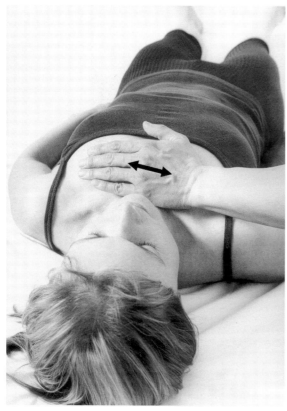

Fig. 4.2

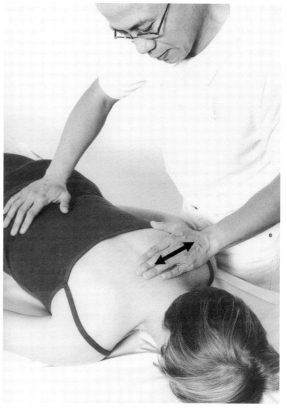

Fig. 4.3

Rou 揉 **Kneading**

- With the thumb
- Stand at the head of the table and perform slow circular movements with the thumb 0.5 *cun* on both sides from the spinous process of C7; 1 minute.
- EX-17
→ **Fig. 4.4**

Rou 揉 **Kneading**

- With the thumbs
- On BL-13 on both sides
- Three minutes

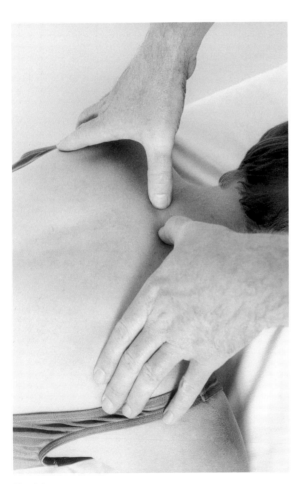

Fig. 4.4

Tui 推 Pushing

- With the thumbs placed on top of each other
- In supine position on the sternum from the manubrium to the xiphoid
- Three to five times each in the exhalatory phase

→ **Fig. 4.5**

Fen Tui 分推 Lateral Pushing

- With the thumbs
- Palpate the intercostal space on both sides and then push symmetrically from the sternum to lateral. Beginning with intercostal space 1–2 and successively up to intercostal space 7–8, perform one push each on both sides.
- Three to five passes

→ **Fig. 4.6**

Rou 揉 Kneading

- With the thumb with gentle pressure
- In supine position
- CV-22
- CV-17
- Five minutes each

For Symptoms of Vacuity

An 按 Pressing

- With the thumb
- On the seated patient
- ST-36
- KI-3

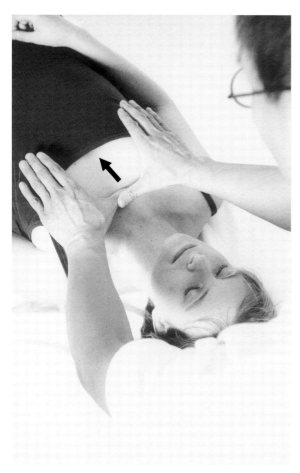

Fig. 4.5

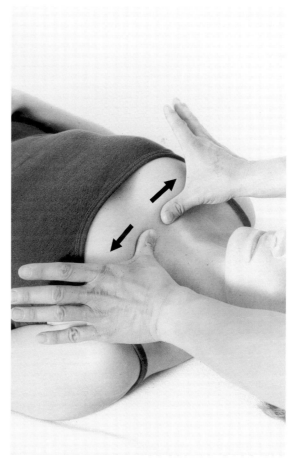

Fig. 4.6

An 按 **Pressing**

- In prone position
- BL-23

For Symptoms of Repletion

An 按 **Pressing**

- With the thumb
- On the seated patient
- LI-4
- ST-40
- The points can be pressed simultaneously on both sides; up to 1 minute.

Arterial Hypertension

Symptoms of Vacuity

Headache, dizziness, tinnitus, forgetfulness, internal restlessness, restless dreams, feeling of weakness in the legs and sore muscles in the back, fatigue, shortness of breath.

Symptoms of Repletion

Headache, dizziness, red face, inflamed edges of the eyelids, easily irritated, rage, bitter taste in the mouth, solid stools, feeling of heaviness in the head.

General Treatment

An 按 **Pressing**

- LI-11
- SI-8
- ST-36

Tui 推 **Pushing**

- With the balls of the hands
- Bladder channel on both sides from the neck to the foot
- Three to five times
→ See **Fig. 2.19a–d** in Chapter 2

Na 拿 **Grasping**

- On the seated patient
- With both hands
- Use the pinch grip to slowly pull up a bulge above the horizontal trapezius and release, on both sides.
- Up to three times on each side
→ **Fig. 4.7**

Mo Fu 摩腹 **Round-rubbing the Abdomen**

- In supine position
- In clockwise direction; 5–10 minutes

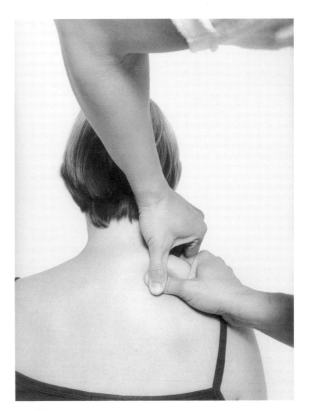

Fig. 4.7

Qian Yin 牵引 Traction

- In supine position
- On fingers and toes on both sides
- Once each
→ **Fig. 4.8a, b**

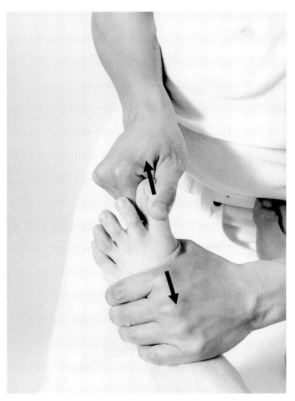

Fig. 4.8a

For Symptoms of Vacuity

An 按 Pressing

- SP-6
- KI-3
- CV-6
- CV-3

For Symptoms of Repletion

An 按 Pressing

- LR-3
- PC-6
- ST-40

Reflux Esophagitis, Gastritis, Attendant Treatment of Ulcer Disorders

Symptoms of Vacuity

Pulling pain in the upper abdomen; on the location of the discomfort, the practitioner's hand is experienced as comforting; drafts and cold aggravate the pain; soft stools and diarrhea, internal restlessness, dry mouth, moist palms of the hands and soles of the feet.

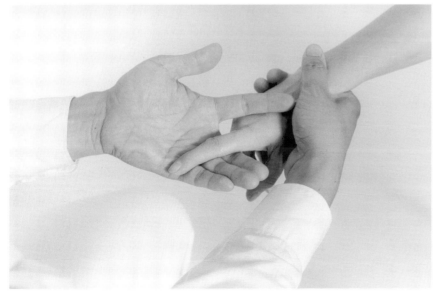

Fig. 4.8b

Symptoms of Repletion

Upper abdominal pain with feeling of distention and pulling pain below the costal arches, acid reflux with belching, heart burn; pain that is also related to anger and is aggravated by excitement and anger; drinking cold fluids relieves the pain; dry mouth and bad breath, solid stools.

General Treatment

Tui 推 **Pushing**

- With the balls of the hands
- In prone position, on both sides
- On top of the bladder channel from the lower cervical spine to the sacrum
- Five times
- → **Fig. 4.9**

Rou 揉 **Kneading**

- With the balls of the hands
- In prone position

- Simultaneously on both sides on top of the bladder channels, descending from the area of the middle thoracic spine to the lower lumbar spine
- Three to five passes
- → See **Fig. 1.8** in Chapter 1

For Symptoms of Vacuity

An 按 **Pressing**

- BL-18
- BL-21

Rou 揉 **Kneading**

- With the thumb
- In supine position
- CV-4
- ST-41
- SP-6

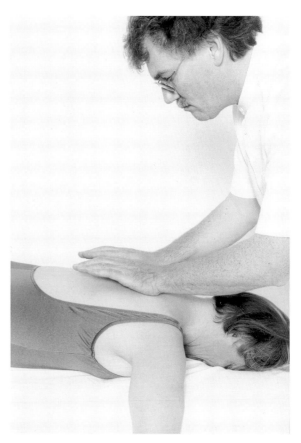

Fig. 4.9

For Symptoms of Repletion

An 按 **Pressing**

- In supine position
- LR-3
- CV-6

Fen Tui 分推 **Lateral Pushing**

- With the ball of the hand
- In prone or seated position
- Stroke simultaneously on both sides on top of the ribs laterally, from the upper thoracic spine section to the lumbar spine; 3 minutes.
- → **Fig. 4.10**

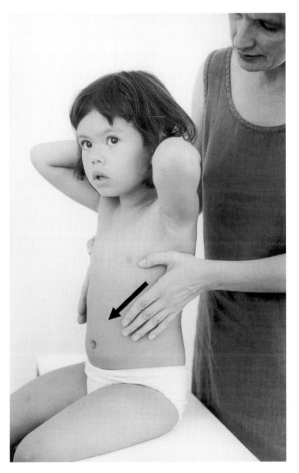

Fig. 4.10

Constipation

Symptoms of Vacuity

Weak constitution in elderly patients, lusterless skin and lips, psychological exhaustion with fatigue, no strength to push, soft stools.

Symptoms of Repletion

Dry mouth, bad breath, concentrated urine, feeling of tension under the costal arch, shortness of breath, solid stools.

General Treatment

An 按 Pressing

- ST-25
- ST-37
- BL-25

Tui 推 Pushing

- In prone position
- Descending on the bladder channel from the neck to the foot
- Three to five times
- → See **Fig. 2.19a–d** in Chapter 2

Mo Fu 摩腹 Round-rubbing the Abdomen

- In supine position
- With the flat hand
- In clockwise and counterclockwise direction for 5–10 minutes
- → **Fig. 4.11**

For Symptoms of Vacuity

An 按 Pressing

- BL-20, BL-21
- CV-6

For Symptoms of Repletion

An 按 Pressing

- TB-5
- LI-11

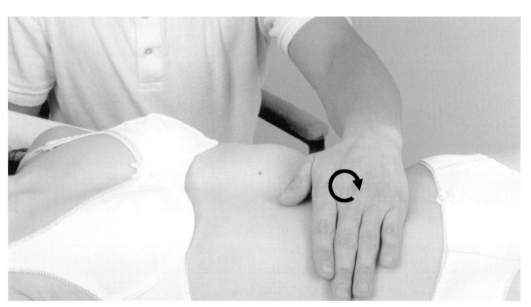

Fig. 4.11

Urinary Tract Infections, Attendant Treatment of Cystitis, of Pyelonephritis, and of Incontinence and its Prevention

Symptoms of Vacuity

Frequent urinary urgency and feeling of incomplete voiding of the bladder, urinary urgency that increases with physical exertion, feeling of weakness in the back, dizziness, tinnitus, forgetfulness, restlessness, irritability, sleep disorders, dry mouth, pale facial complexion, soft stools, tendency to cold hands, cold feet.

Symptoms of Repletion

Frequent urination with pain, intense yellow coloration of the urine, feeling of warmth in the body, feeling of tension and pain in the lower abdomen, dry mouth, solid stools.

General Treatment

An 按 Pressing

- BL-23
- BL-28

Rou 揉 Kneading

- With the thumb
- CV-3
- SP-6
- Three to 5 minutes each

Tui 推 Pushing

 or

Rou 揉 Kneading

- With the balls of the hands
- In prone position
- On both sides on the bladder channel, descending from the upper lumbar spine to the sacrum
- Three to five times
→ See **Fig. 4.9**

For Symptoms of Vacuity

An 按 Pressing

- With the thumb
- CV-6
- ST-36
- LI-4

For Symptoms of Repletion

An 按 Pressing

- TB-5
- LR-3
- SP-9

Psychovegetative Stress Symptoms, Exhaustion

Symptoms of Vacuity

Insomnia, easily woken up, lots of dreams, tachycardia, forgetfulness, dizziness, tinnitus, feeling of sore muscles in the back, tired legs.

Symptoms of Repletion

Symptoms of repletion are not considered relevant to this disorder.

An 按 Pressing

- In prone position
- GB-20
- GB-21
- SI-14
- SI-11
- BL-15
- BL-20
- BL-23

Shu Ca 竖擦 **Longitudinal Scrubbing**

- In prone position
- On the skin along the longitudinal axis above the sacrum until a feeling of warmth appears; approximately 1 minute
→ **Fig. 4.12**

Tui 推 **Pushing**

- With the thumbs on the head, alternatively with the balls of the hands, on both sides five to eight times
- In prone position on the bladder channel, from the area of the apex to the foot
→ See **Fig. 2.19a–d** in Chapter 2

An 按 **Pressing**

- In supine position
- EX-2 (*tai yang*) on both sides

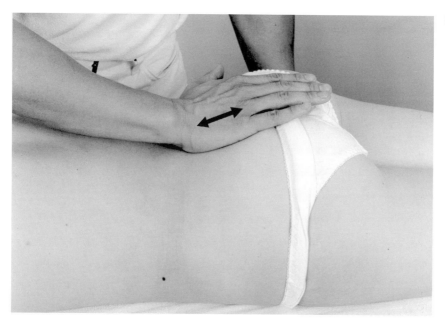

Fig. 4.12

An 按 **Pressing**

- In supine position
- Position the fingers of each hand in opposition to each other. Now slowly press down with the tips and finger nails with both hands simultaneously, in different locations on the scalp, whereby the finger tips should press into the scalp as vertically as possible.
- Avoid clawing into the skin with the nails; 2 minutes.
→ **Fig. 4.13**

Mo Fu 摩腹 **Round-rubbing the Abdomen**

- In supine position
- Slowly in clockwise direction with the flat hand; 5–10 minutes
→ See **Fig. 4.11**

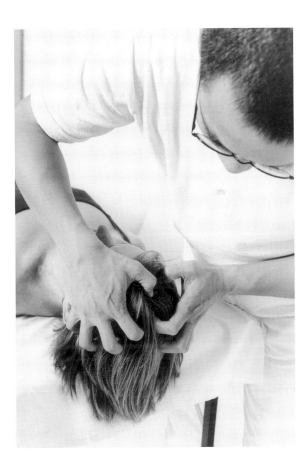

Fig. 4.13

Sleeping Disorders

Symptoms of Vacuity

Many dreams, easily woken up, tachycardia, forgetfulness, dizziness, tinnitus, pensiveness, feeling of sore muscles in the back, tired legs.

Symptoms of Repletion

Headache, dizziness, feeling of tension below the costal arch, irritability, enraged mood, belching, and feeling of fullness.

General Treatment

An 按 **Pressing**

- HT-7
- SP-6
- EX-1 (*yin tang*)
- EX-5 (*an mian*) between GB-20 and TB-17

Mo Fu 摩腹 **Round-rubbing the Abdomen**

- With the flat hand
- In supine position
- In clockwise direction in concert with breathing, stroking upward on the right during inhalation and stroking downward on the left during exhalation
- Ten times
→ See **Fig. 4.11**

Tui 推 **Pushing**

- With the ball of the hand
- In prone position
- On the bladder channel on both sides from the neck down to the foot
- Three to five times
→ See **Fig. 2.19a–d** in Chapter 2

For Symptoms of Vacuity

An 按 **Pressing**

- BL-15
- BL-19
- BL-20, BL-23
- KI-3

For Symptoms of Repletion

An 按 Pressing

- BL-18
- BL-21
- LR-3
- ST-36

Headache

Symptoms of Vacuity

Diffuse headache, headache aggravated by physical exertion, lusterless face, sensitivity to cold.

Symptoms of Repletion

Easily localizable pain, strong sensitivity to pain, red face and a bitter taste in the mouth, irritability, rage, dizziness.

General Treatment

Tui 推 Pushing

- With the ball of the hand
- In lying or sitting position
- On the bladder channel from the neck to the sacrum
- Three to five times
- → **Fig. 4.14**

> ❗ We especially recommend treatment in the sitting position, whereby you can prop the elbow against the iliac crest to increase the push at the height of the thoracic and lumbar spine.

Na 拿 Grasping

- With both hands
- Area of the trapezius and splenius cervicis on both sides
- Three to five times
- → **Fig. 4.15**

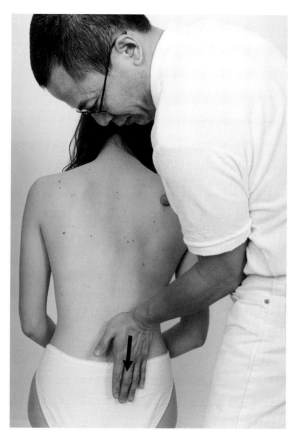

Fig. 4.14

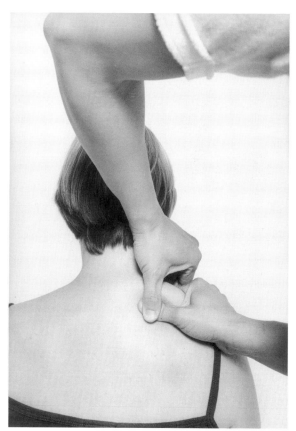

Fig. 4.15

For Symptoms of Vacuity

An 按 **Pressing**

- CV-4
- ST-36

Mo Fu 摩腹 **Round-rubbing the Abdomen**

- In supine position
- With the flat hand
- In clockwise direction; 3–5 minutes

For Symptoms of Repletion

An 按 **Pressing**

- LR-3
- GB-43

Frontal Headache

An 按 **Pressing**

- EX-1 (*yin tang*) between the eyebrows
- GV-23

Tui 推 **Pushing**

- With the tips of both thumbs in alternating rhythm
- From EX-1 (*yin tang*) to the frontal hairline
- Five to 10 times
- → **Fig. 4.16**

Fen Tui 分推 **Lateral Pushing**

- With the thumbs
- From the middle of the forehead to the area of the temples. Begin on the eyebrows and then move in sections of about 1 cm each cranially, up to the frontal hairline.
- Three to five passes
- → **Fig. 4.17**

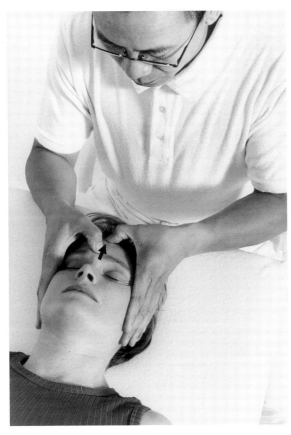

Fig. 4.16

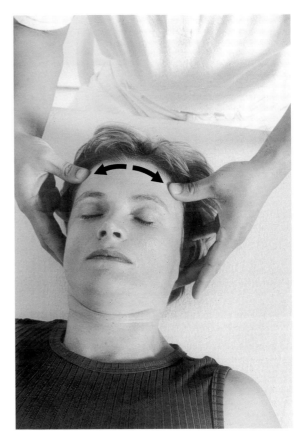

Fig. 4.17

Lateral Headache, Temple Headache

An 按 **Pressing**

- GB-20
- TB-5

Tui 推 **Pushing**

- With the radial edge of the thumb
- Beginning approximately 4 cm above the EX-2 (*tai yang*), toward this point
- Slow pushing up to five times
- → **Fig. 4.18**

Gua 刮 **Scratching**

- The tips of fingers 2 to 5 (with short nails) approach the scalp vertically and stroke the gallbladder channel and its vicinity in front of, on top of, and behind the ears.
- Three to five times
- → **Fig. 4.19**

An 按 **Pressing**

- In supine position
- Repeatedly press with the tips of all fingers (with clipped nails) on the scalp in the area of the temples, in different locations.
- Slowly increase the pressure, hold for 3–5 seconds, and release.
- Three to five times

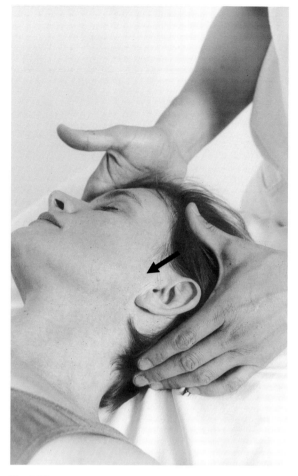

Fig. 4.18

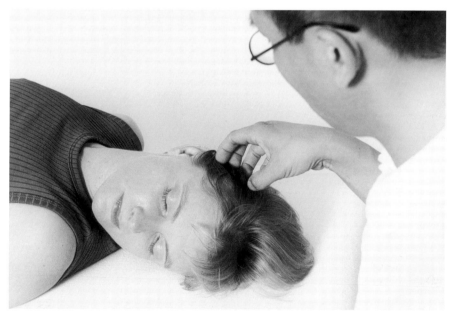

Fig. 4.19

Occipital Headache

An 按 **Pressing**

or

Rou 揉 **Kneading**

- GV-19
- GB-20
- BL-9, BL-10
- EX-2 (*tai yang*)
- SI-3

Fen Tui 分推 **Lateral Pushing**

- In supine position
- With the tips of the thumbs on the eyebrows
- Five to 10 times
- → **Fig. 4.20**

Fen Tui 分推 **Lateral Pushing**

- With the thumbs with only mild pressure on the closed upper eyelids
- Three times
- → **Fig. 4.21**

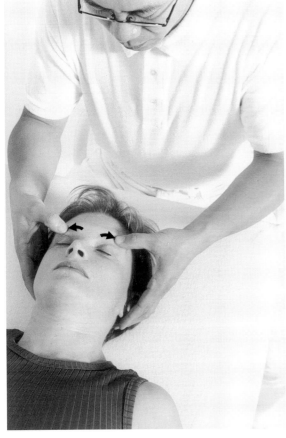

Fig. 4.20

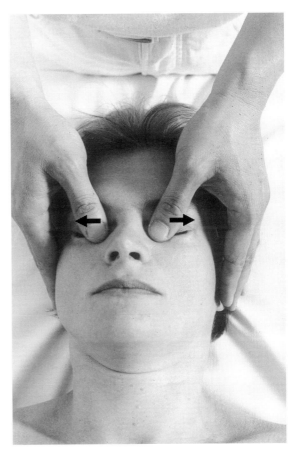

Fig. 4.21

Vertex Headache

An 按 **Pressing**

- GV-20
- BL-7 on both sides
- LR-2
- KI-1

An 按 **Pressing**

- In supine position
- Repeatedly press with the tips of all fingers on the scalp in the area of the vertex, in different locations.
- Slowly increase the pressure, hold for 3–5 seconds, and release.
- Three to five times

→ **Fig. 4.22**

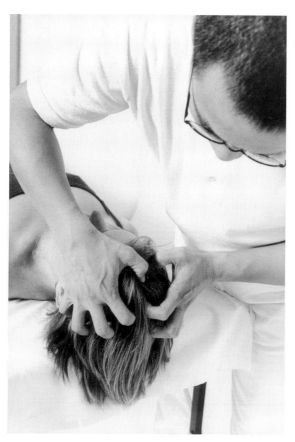

Fig. 4.22

5 Gynecological and Obstetric Indications

Menstrual Irregularities, Delayed or Early Menstruation

Symptoms of Vacuity

Tendency to delayed menstruation, scant amount, weak blood color, thin consistency, pale facial complexion, fatigue, lack of strength, tachycardia and dizziness, weakness and soreness in the back, weak legs, reduced appetite, soft stools.

Symptoms of Repletion

Early onset of menstruation, dark red blood color, thick consistency, red face, red lips, abdominal pain, dry mouth.

General Treatment

Heng Ca 橫擦 **Transverse Scrubbing**

- With the flat hand
- In prone position
- Rapid rubbing on top of the sacrum
- One hundred to 200 times
- → **Fig. 5.1**

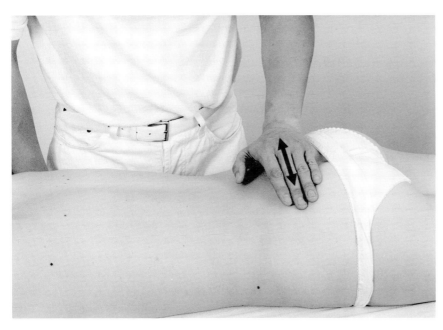

Fig. 5.1

Shu Ca 竖擦   **Longitudinal Scrubbing**

- With the flat hand
- In supine position
- On the inner thighs on both sides at medium speed; 1 minute each
→ **Fig. 5.2**

Tui Liang Lei 推两肋   **Pushing the Ribs on Both Sides**

- With the balls of the hands
- In seated position
- Stand behind the patient.
- Push from the lateral thorax to the middle and lower abdomen on both sides; up to 3 minutes.
→ See **Fig. 4.10** in Chapter 4

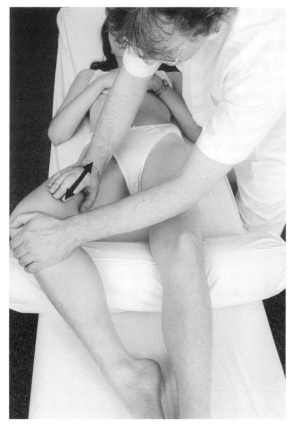

Fig. 5.2

For Symptoms of Vacuity

An 按   **Pressing**

- CV-6
- ST-36
- LI-4
- BL-23

For Symptoms of Repletion

An 按   **Pressing**

- SP-10
- LR-3
- SP-6
- CV-3

Abnormally Painful Menstruation

Symptoms of Vacuity

Regular onset, painful, mild pain, indeterminate pain, fatigue, pale facial complexion; cold hands, cold feet, soft stools.

Symptoms of Repletion

The abdomen is taut and very painful, pain to below the costal arches, sensitivity to touch, dark blood, clotted consistency, feeling of relief after discharge of clots, dry mouth, no thirst, solid stools.

General Treatment

An 按   **Pressing**

- CV-3
- SP-6
- LV-3

For Symptoms of Vacuity

An 按   **Pressing**

- ST-36
- BL-23
- BL-20
- GV-4

For Symptoms of Repletion

An 按   **Pressing**

- SP-10
- BL-32

Amenorrhea

Symptoms of Vacuity

Cold hands, cold feet, pale appearance, headache, dizziness, general exhaustion, shortness of breath.

Symptoms of Repletion

Dark red face, dry skin, scaly skin, dry mouth, no thirst, taut painful abdomen, sensitive to touch, solid stools.

General Treatment

An 按 Pressing

- CV-3
- SP-6

Tui An 推按 Transverse Rubbing

- With flat hands
- In supine position
- On the abdomen at medium speed rhythmically in opposite directions, for about 2 minutes

→ **Fig. 5.3**

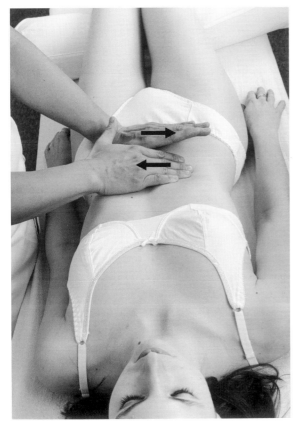

Fig. 5.3

Na 拿 Grasping

- With both hands
- In supine position
- From the lower abdomen to the upper abdomen, grasp the horizontal folds of the abdominal wall approximately 10 times and pull up, hold for 2–3 seconds, and let go.
- Up to two passes
→ **Fig. 5.4**

For Symptoms of Vacuity

An 按 Pressing

- ST-36
- BL-23
- CV-6
- CV-17

For Symptoms of Repletion

An 按 Pressing

- SP-10
- LR-2

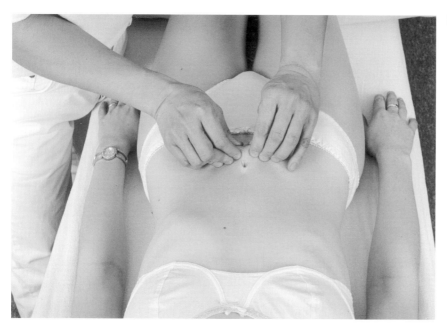

Fig. 5.4

Obstetrical Measures in the Delivery Ward when Post-term

Symptoms of Vacuity

General feeling of weakness, pale face, exhaustion, tachycardia, shortness of breath.

Symptoms of Repletion

Nervousness, depressed mood, pensiveness, strong abdominal pain, discomfort in the thorax.

General Treatment

Shu Ca 竖擦 Longitudinal Scrubbing

- With the ball of the hand
- On the seated patient
- On the sacrum at medium speed, only rubbing caudally; 10 minutes
- → **Fig. 5.5**

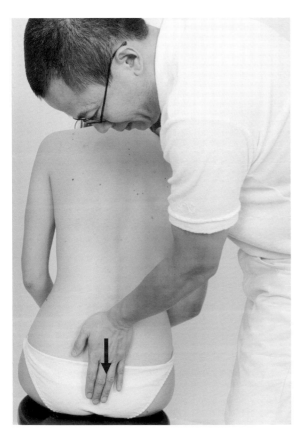

Fig. 5.5

For Symptoms of Vacuity

An 按 Pressing

- ST-36
- SP-10

For Symptoms of Repletion

An 按 Pressing

- LI-4
- SP-6
- BL-67

Scant or Lacking Lactation

Symptoms of Vacuity

Scant milk, thin consistency, pale face, dull skin, dizziness, tinnitus, tachycardia, shortness of breath, no appetite, soft stools.

Symptoms of Repletion

Tautness in the chest, swelling and pain in the chest, discomfort in the costal arch, distention, lack of appetite, feeling of cold or heat.

General Treatment

An 按 Pressing

- CV-17
- ST-18

For Symptoms of Vacuity

An 按 Pressing

- BL-20
- ST-36

For Symptoms of Repletion

An 按 Pressing

- BL-18
- SP-6
- SI-1

6 Self-treatment for Adults

Lack of Concentration, Fatigued Vision

An 按 **Pressing**

- In pinch grip between thumb and index finger
- BL-1 at the level of the bridge of the nose, slightly medial to the inner canthus
- Slowly increase the pressure and then release it.
- Three to five times
→ **Fig. 6.1**

Rou 揉 **Kneading**

- With index or middle fingers
- Between ST-2 and ST-3 at the same time centrally on the cheeks; approximately 1 minute
→ **Fig. 6.2**

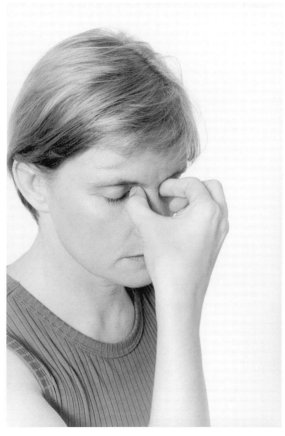

Fig. 6.1

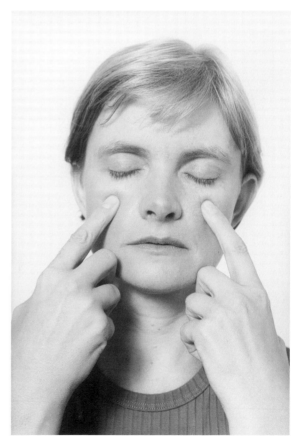

Fig. 6.2

Rou 揉 **Kneading**

- With the tips of the thumbs
- In seated position
- On the medial beginnings of the eyebrows (BL-2). With hands folded, place the tips of the thumbs on both sides simultaneously on the points.

- With gentle pressure, slowly perform small circling movements with the eyes closed; 3–5 minutes.
→ **Fig. 6.3**

Fig. 6.3

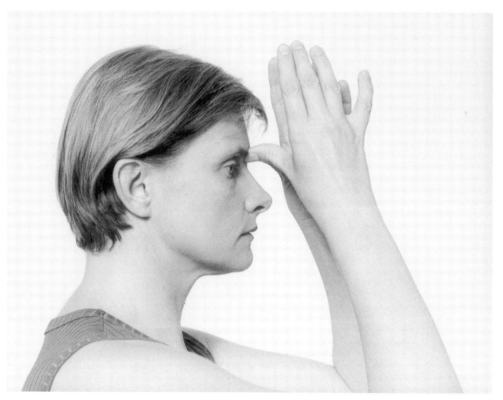

An 按 **Pressing**

and

Rou 揉 **Kneading**

- With the tips of the thumbs
- Place the fingers, spread apart, onto the back of the head and push with the tips of the thumbs on the appropriate points in the muscle attachments of the proximal neck area.
- Hereby, you can also perform circling movements.
- Pressing is also effective if you lay the head slowly and rhythmically back into the neck while maintaining the pressure on GB-20. Movements dorsally at an approximately 20° angle.
- Total duration of treatment *rou* 2 or 3 minutes, *an* two to four treatment rhythms in combination of acupressure with backward tilt of the head.

→ **Fig. 6.4**

An 按 **Pressing**

and

Tui 推 **Pushing**

- In seated position
- Place the thumb on EX-2 (*tai yang*) on both sides. Use the radial edge of the middle phalanx of the index finger to work the eyebrow symmetrically from medial to lateral in 2- or 3-second intervals with medium or slightly stronger pressure. Alternating every 30 seconds, also stroke with the edge of the index finger in the same way on the upper cheek section from medial to lateral. The thumb pressure remains on EX-2.
- Total duration of treatment 3–5 minutes

→ **Fig. 6.5a, c**

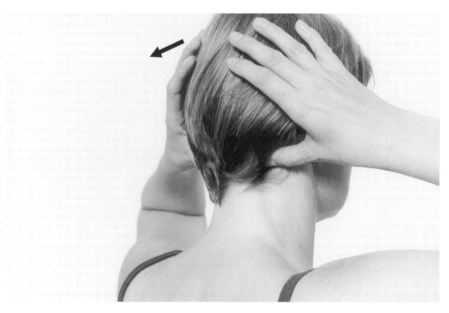

Fig. 6.4

Lateral or Frontal Headache

Tui 推 **Pushing**

- Place the tips of the thumbs on EX-2 (*tai yang*), on the frontal section of the temples. With the radial edges of the middle phalanges of the index fingers, stroke from medial to lateral on both sides on the eyebrows, then on the forehead above the eyebrows, and lastly on the upper cheek section.
- Three to five times each
→ **Fig. 6.5a–c**

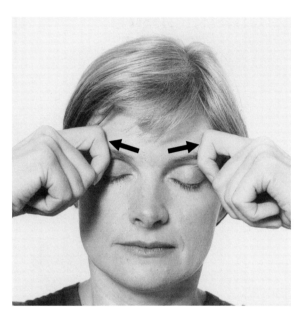

Fig. 6.5a

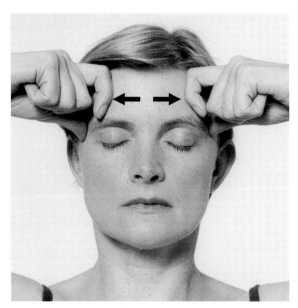

Fig. 6.5b

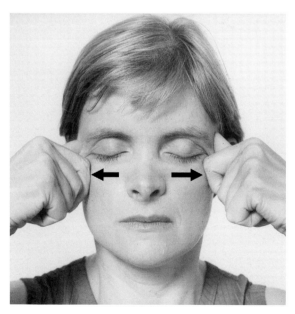

Fig. 6.5c

Shoulder and Arm Pain

Na 拿 **Grasping**

- With the opposite hand, grasp the top of the shoulder. Without involving the thumb, the other four fingers and the palm grip the horizontal section of the trapezius, pull it up, and abruptly let go.
- Three to five times
→ **Fig. 6.6**

An 按 **Pressing**

- With the index and middle fingers of the opposite hand, grasp the shoulder that you want to treat.
- Index and middle finger push on SI-10 above the dorsal edge of the glenoidal labrum.
→ **Fig. 6.7**

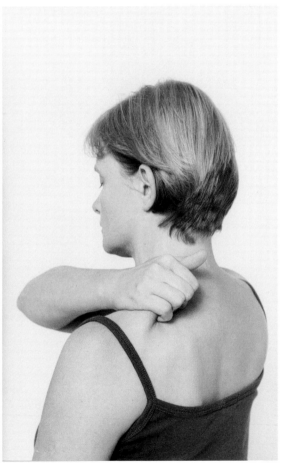

Fig. 6.6

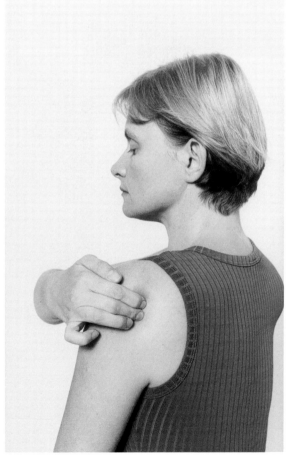

Fig. 6.7

An 按 **Pressing**

- With the index or middle finger on TB-14, to the side of the lateral edge of the acromion
- Build pressure slowly and release two times.

→ **Fig. 6.8**

> **!** Slightly dorsal or ventral from TB-14, you can also localize a trigger point that is treated in the same way. In cases with isolated shoulder pain, you can use this technique alone.

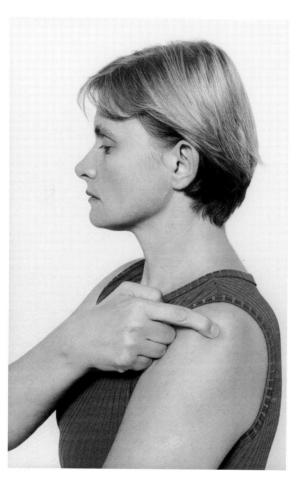

Fig. 6.8

Shoulder and Arm Pain with Neck Pain and Occipital Headache

An 按 **Pressing**

and

Rou 揉 **Kneading**

- With the tips of the thumbs on GB-20 and BL-10
- Place the fingers, spread apart, on the back of the head and push with the tips of the thumbs on the appropriate points in the muscle attachments of the proximal neck area.

- Hereby, you can also perform circling movements (*rou*).
- Pressing (*an*) is also effective if you lay the head slowly and rhythmically back into the neck while maintaining the pressure on GB-20 and BL-10.
- Movements dorsally at an approximately 20° angle. Total duration of treatment *rou* 2 or 3 minutes, *an* two to four treatment rhythms in combination with acupressure with backward tilt of the head.

→ **Fig. 6.9a, b**

! You can use this technique exclusively for occipital headache.

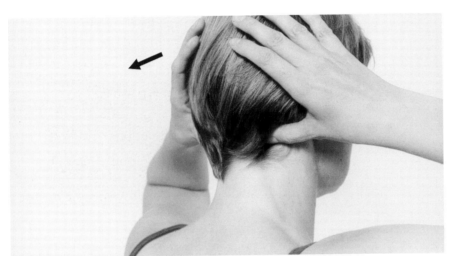

Fig. 6.9a

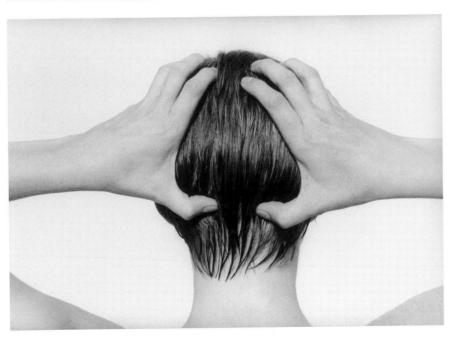

Fig. 6.9b

Rou 揉 **Kneading**

- With the thumb
- Slow circling movements on the intermediate part of the deltoid, descending from the acromion to the attachment and then on distally between biceps and triceps in the direction of the elbow
- Work this stretch two or three times in succession.

→ **Fig. 6.10**

- In the same way, with circling pushing movements of the thumb in opposition to the four fingers, two or three times.

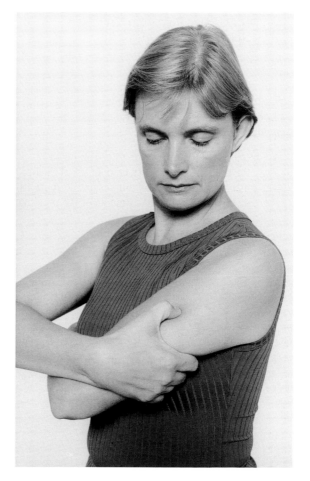

Fig. 6.10

Qian Yin 牵引 **Traction**

- The opposite hand grips the distal section of the forearm from dorsal.
- With the arm raised forward at 60–70°, cause a horizontal adduction and pull on the shoulder. Slowly build the pull, hold for 2 or 3 seconds, and release.
- As an alternative, you can also perform this exercise against a doorframe.

→ **Fig. 6.11a, b**

! Carefully regulate the stretch!

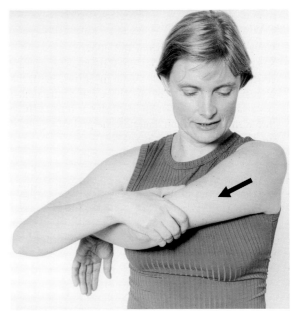

Fig. 6.11a

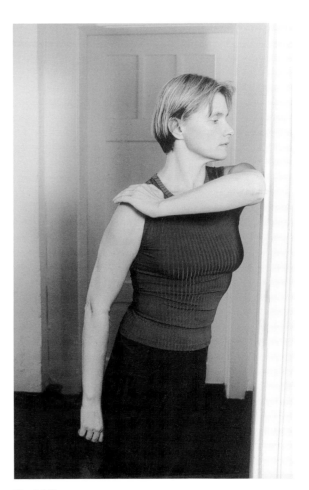

Fig. 6.11b

Qian Yin 牵引 **Traction**

- Forced stretching by clasping the elbow
- Raise the arm in the shoulder laterally as far as possible, with the elbow in maximum flexion. With the opposite hand, clasp the distal section of the dorsal upper arm or the wrist and pull the arm from there into a small extension. Increase the pull slowly, hold for 2 or 3 seconds, and release.

→ **Fig. 6.12**

! Carefully regulate the stretch!

Rou 揉 **Kneading**

- GB-34 at the head of the fibula
- One minute

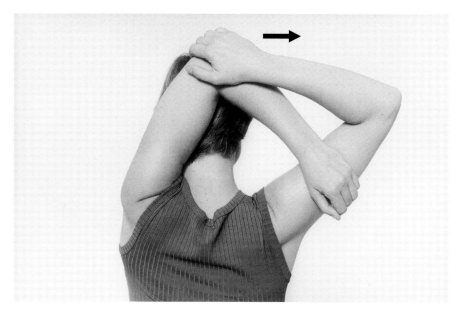

Fig. 6.12

Pain in the Area of the Lumbar Spine, Pain in the Sacrum

Rou 揉 Kneading

- With the tips of the thumbs
- On the eye points of the back
- Hereby, the four fingers support themselves on both sides on the flanks, and the tip of the thumb pushes into the lateral edge of the lumbar bulge roughly at the level of L3/4. Perform slow circling movements with the greatest possible pressure; up to 1 minute.

Tui 推 Pushing

- With the balls of the hands
- Place the hands bilaterally on the paravertebral area, with the fingers pointing down. The movement runs from the lowest ribs down to the sacroiliac joints.
- Three to five times
→ **Fig. 6.13a, b**

Mo Fu 摩腹 Round-rubbing the Abdomen

- With hands placed on top of each other, perform slow circling movements in clockwise direction.
- Slowly inhale during the upstroke and exhale while moving downward on the left side of the abdomen.
- Duration of treatment 3–5 minutes

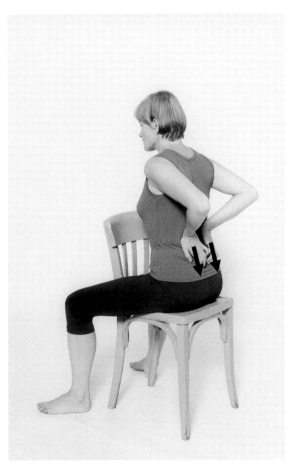

Fig. 6.13a

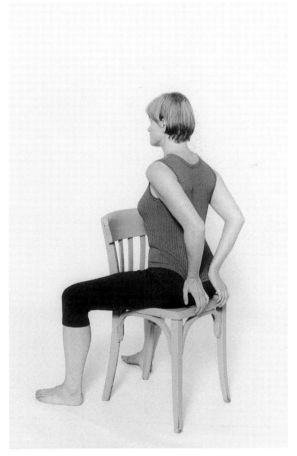

Fig. 6.13b

Combination of

Rou 揉 **Kneading**

and

Tui 推 **Pushing**

- With the gripping surface of the thumb
- GB-34 on the head of the fibula for about 20 seconds, then slowly push downward on both sides on the lateral edge of the fibula to the ankle.
- Combination three to five times
→ **Fig. 6.14**

Xuan Zhuan Fa 旋转法 **Rotating Mobilization of the Ankle**

- In seated position
- Place the lower leg of the treatment side crosswise on top of the other leg's thigh. One hand clasps the leg above the ankle area. The other clasps the forefoot from plantar and carries out circling movements in clockwise and counterclockwise direction.
- Three to five times per side
→ **Fig. 6.15**

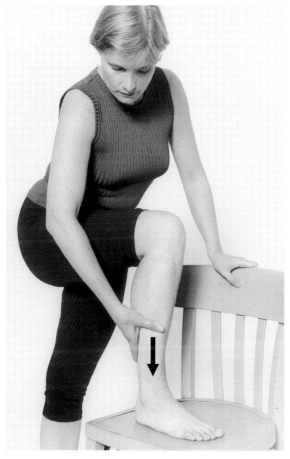

Fig. 6.14

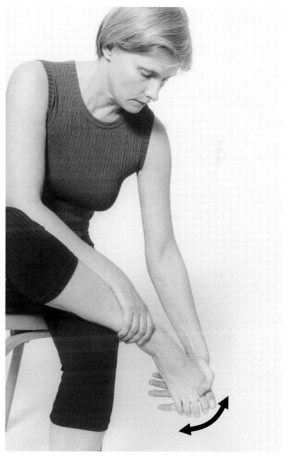

Fig. 6.15

Knee Pain

Tui 推 Pushing

- With the balls of the hands
- In seated position, with the knees flexed at right angles
- With short strong pushes, descending on the medial and lateral part of the proximal ventral recess of the knee joint on both sides from the quadriceps attachment. The pushes follow the stomach channel laterally in the vicinity of ST-34.
- Three to 5 minutes
→ **Fig. 6.16**

Rou 揉 Kneading

- With the ball of the hand in clockwise and counter-clockwise direction
- On top of the distal quadriceps attachment proximal to the patella
- Two or 3 minutes
→ **Fig. 6.17**

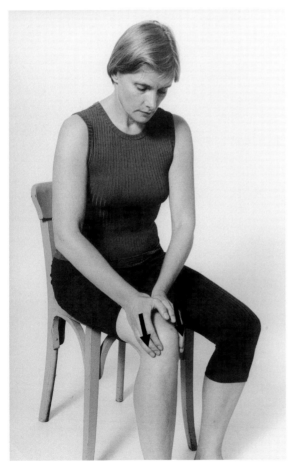

Fig. 6.16

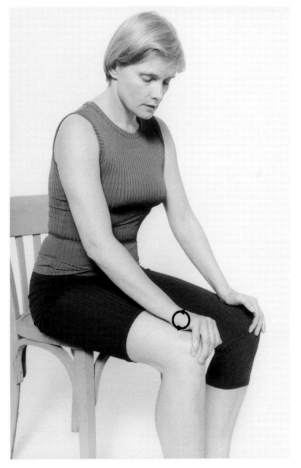

Fig. 6.17

An 按 Pressing

- With the thumb
- In seated position with the knee joint slightly flexed (20–30°)
- Pressure on the lateral and medial eye points of the knee (see also p. 72 f) on the Hoffa fat pad.
- Slowly increase the pressure, hold for 3 seconds, and then release.
- Three to five times

→ **Fig. 6.18**

An 按 Pressing

- GB-34

and subsequently

Tui 推 Pushing

- With the thumb
- On top of the distal part of the gallbladder channel down to the exterior ankle
- Two or three times
- Accompanied by circling mobilization of the ankle as described above

→ See **Figs. 6.14** and **6.15**

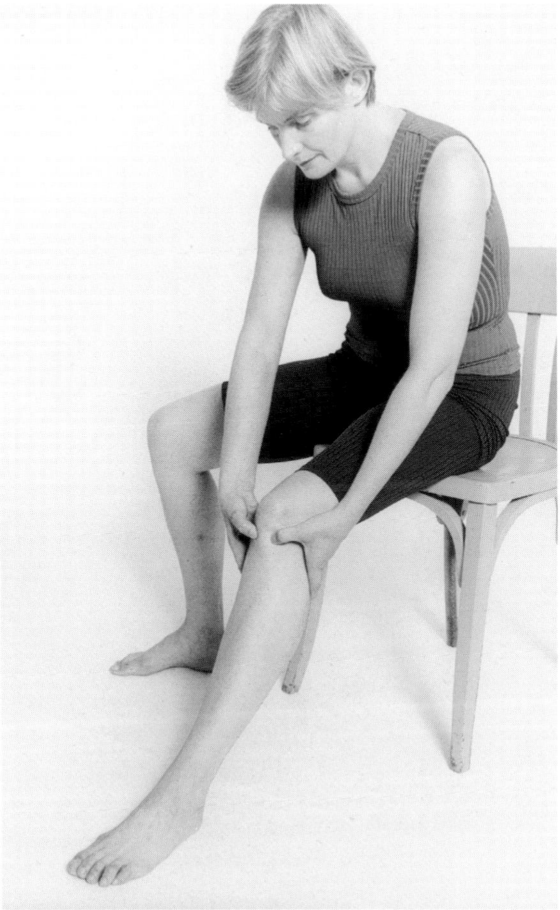

Fig. 6.18

Gastrointestinal Complaints

Tui 推 **Pushing**

- With the arms bent by the side of the body, place the hands with the ball of the little finger on the lower lateral rib section. The fingers point to the navel.
- Push with strong symmetrical movements downward across the lateral and frontal costal arch toward the upper abdomen.
- Three to five times
→ **Fig. 6.19**

Tui 推 **Pushing**

- With the wrist
- From the lateral rib section with forward- and downward-pointing movements to the navel and to the lower abdomen
- Three to five times
→ **Fig. 6.20**

Mo Fu 摩腹 **Round-rubbing the Abdomen**

- With hands placed on top of each other
- In clockwise direction, perform spacious circling movements on the abdomen in concert with your breathing rhythm, that is, inhaling during the upstroke on the right side of the abdomen and exhaling during the downstroke on the left.
- Three to 5 minutes

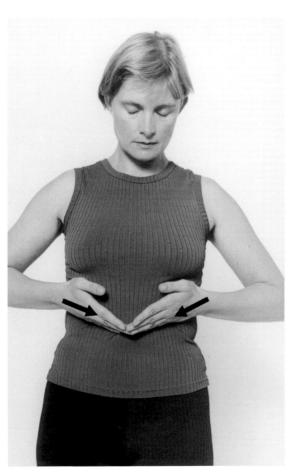

Fig. 6.19

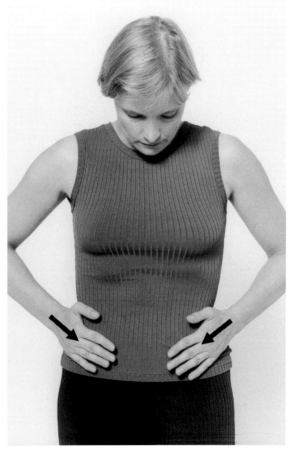

Fig. 6.20

Tui 推 **Pushing**

- With the balls of the hands
- Slowly descending on both sides from the lower rib section on top of the psoas bulge down to the iliosacral joints

- This technique can also be coordinated with the breathing rhythm, placing the hands cranially on the ribs during inhalation and stroking downward during exhalation.
- Three to five times

→ **Fig. 6.21**

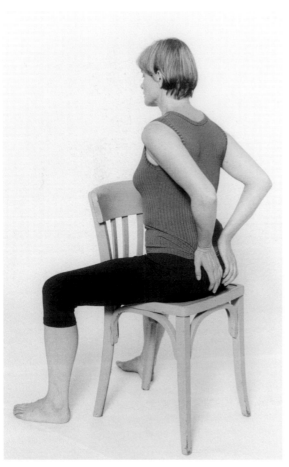

Fig. 6.21

7 Pediatrics

Basic Techniques

Tui 推 Pushing

Modify pushing as in the technique for adults. Push with the tip or gripping surface of the thumb while at the same time positioning three to four fingers for support and fixation (e.g., of the extremity receiving treatment). Alternatively, use the volar surface of the index and middle fingers. The first of these methods, when supported with the other fingers, allows you to carefully regulate the application of force. The frequency should be set markedly higher than in adults, up to 120 per minute (**Fig. 7.1a, b**).

Xuan Tui 旋推 Rotating Pushing

This technique is utilized on the hands and feet of small patients. Use the thumb to perform small circling and rubbing movements with little pressure on the treatment area. Two or three fingers of the same hand serve as a

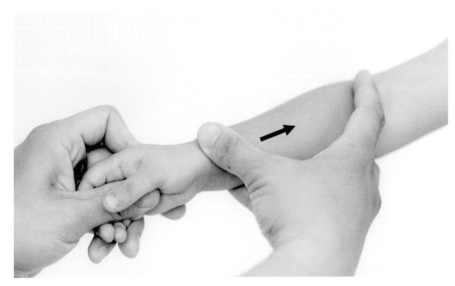

Fig. 7.1a

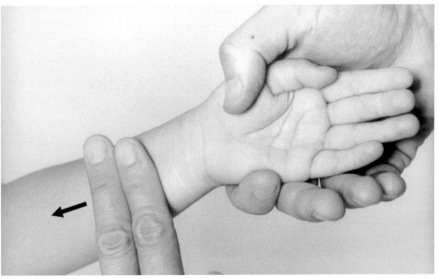

Fig. 7.1b

base to support the treatment object and allow for a very fine regulation of applied force. The movements should be performed with a frequency of 100–200 per minute (**Fig. 7.2**).

Fen Tui 分推   **Lateral Pushing**

In this technique, position the fingers to support the hands and use the thumbs to perform small rhythmic pushing movements that point toward the palm and radial edge of the hand. The treatment frequency should be around 100 per minute (**Fig. 7.3**).

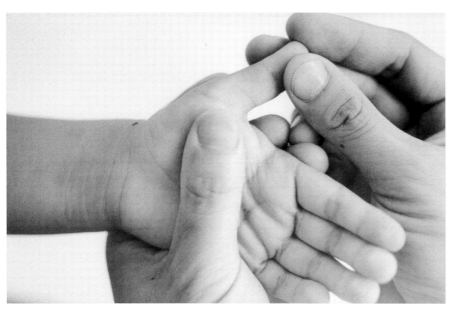

Fig. 7.2

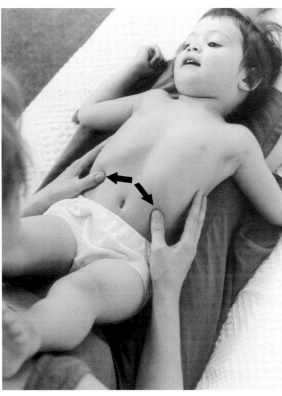

Fig. 7.3

Rou (Dian Rou) 揉（点揉） **Kneading (Point Kneading)**

With the index finger crossed by the middle finger or with the tip of the thumb, perform small circling movements with a frequency of 100–200 per minute.

• CV-17 (**Fig. 7.4a**)

The application of force to the treatment area is greater than in *xuan tui*.

• KI-1 (**Fig. 7.4b**)

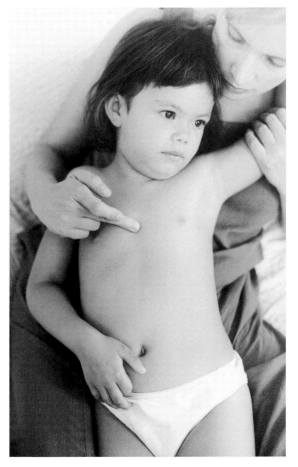

Fig. 7.4a

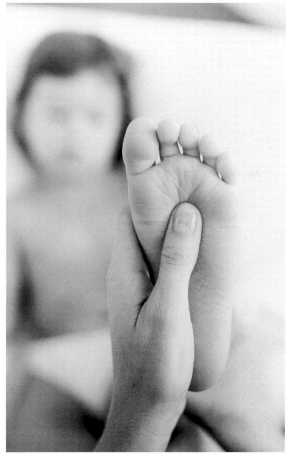

Fig. 7.4b

Na 拿 **Grasping**

As in adults, one time with the three-finger technique in a grip between the thumb and the index and middle fingers or with five fingers. Hereby, it is also possible to apply the grip between the gripping surface of the thumb and the radial edge of the middle phalanx of the index finger (**Fig. 7.5**).

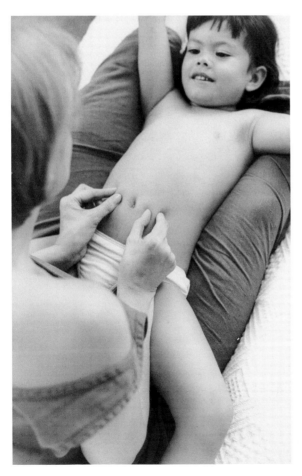

Fig. 7.5

Various Indications

Diarrhea

Symptoms of Vacuity

Mucous stool, pale stool color, not very intense smell, intestinal sounds, abdominal pain, pale facial complexion, no desire for drinks, long-lasting or frequently recurrent diarrhea, often for 2 months, lack of appetite, undigested food particles in the stool.

Symptoms of Repletion

Close link between abdominal pain and diarrhea, explosive diarrhea, intense yellow coloration of stool, stinking stool, dry mouth, desire for drinks, intense yellow urine, bad breath, agitation and crying before the diarrhea, calming down after the diarrhea.

For Symptoms of Vacuity

Xuan Tui (Bu Pi Jing) 旋推　**Rotating Pushing**
（补脾经）　**(Supplementing the Spleen Channel)**

- On the gripping surface of the thumb
- Approximately 100–500 times
→ **Fig. 7.6**

Tui (San Guan) 推（三关）　**Pushing (the Three Bars)**

- With the radial edge of the thumb across the radial side of the thumb proximally. Hereby grasp the distal phalanx of the thumb with two fingers while the active hand pushes with rapid repetitions.
- Approximately 100–500 times
→ **Fig. 7.7**

Tui (Tian He Shui) 推（天和水）　**Pushing (Water from Heaven's River)**

- With two fingers
- On the volar side of the forearm from the wrist to just below the elbow, that is, ascending proximally
- Approximately 100–300 pushes
→ **Fig. 7.8**

Tui (Da Chang) 推（大肠）　**Pushing (the Large Intestine Channel)**

- With the radial edge of the thumb across the gripping surface of the index finger proximally, up to the adduction crease of the thumb
- Approximately 100–300 times
→ **Fig. 7.9**

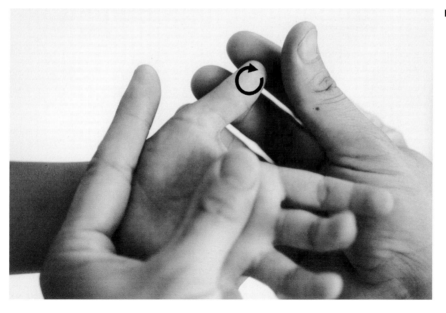

Fig. 7.6

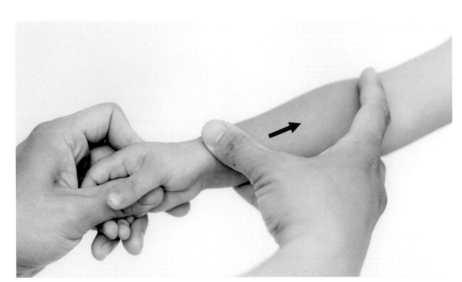

Fig. 7.7

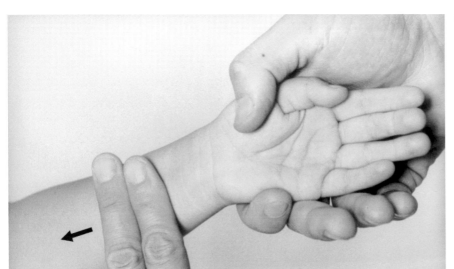

Fig. 7.8

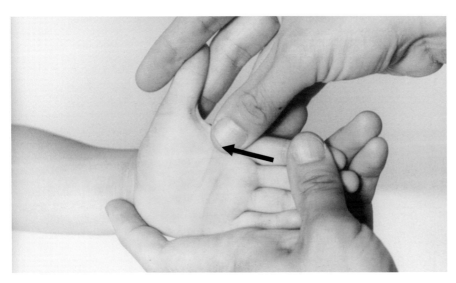

Fig. 7.9

Mo Fu 摩腹   **Round-rubbing the Abdomen**

- Stroke the abdomen in clockwise circling movements with the whole palm of the hand or four fingers.
- Approximately 100–200 times; up to 5 minutes
→ **Fig. 7.10**

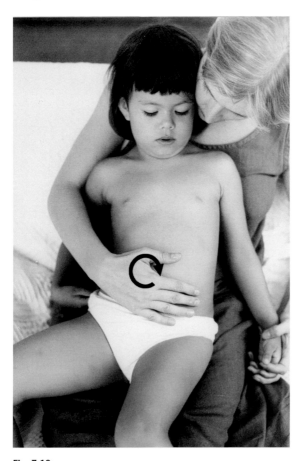

Fig. 7.10

Tui (Qi Jie Gu) 推（七节骨）   **Pushing (the Seventh Vertebra)**

- In prone position
- On the row of spinous processes from the sacrum in the direction of L4 cranially, pushing proximally either with the radial edge of the thumb supported by the other fingers, or with two fingers
- Approximately 100–300 times; 3–5 minutes
→ **Fig. 7.11**

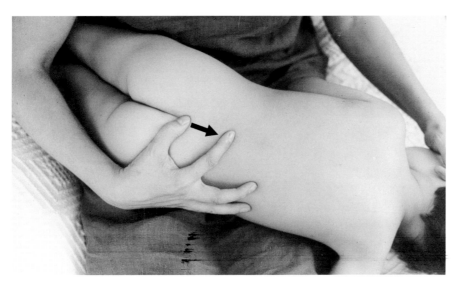

Fig. 7.11

Na (Nie Ji) 拿（捏脊） **Grasping**
(Pinching the Spine)

- In prone position
- Repeatedly grasp and pull the skin parallel to the side of the spinal column in small rolls, ascending from the sacrum. Treatment is upward from the sacrum to the neck.
- Three to five passes
→ **Fig. 7.12**

! The special characteristic of this technique lies in the fact that a skin fold is constantly being lifted up cranially, as a result of which the base layer and skin are continuously rolling through the fingers, while the skin is being grasped and briefly and firmly pulled up once in segments roughly one thumb-width apart, simultaneously on both sides.

For Symptoms of Repletion

Rou (Dian Rou) 揉（点揉） **Kneading**
(Point Kneading)

- With the thumb
- On the gripping surface of the thumb
- Approximately 100–500 times
→ **Fig. 7.13**

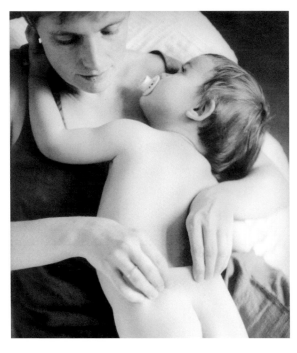

Fig. 7.12

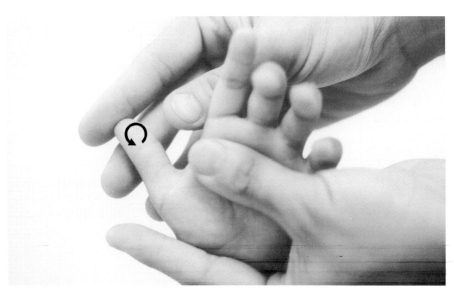

Fig. 7.13

Tui (Qing Da Chang) 推   Pushing
(清大肠) (Cleaning the
Large Intestine)

- With the radial edge of the thumb
- From the transverse crease in the palm distally on the gripping surface of the index finger to the tip
- Approximately 100–500 times
→ **Fig. 7.14**

Tui (Qing Xiao Chang) 推   Pushing
(清小肠) (Cleaning the
Small Intestine)

- With the radial edge of the thumb
- On the ulnar side of the small finger to the tip
- Approximately 100–500 times
→ **Fig. 7.15**

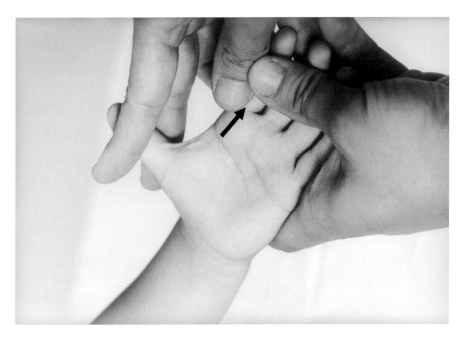

Fig. 7.14

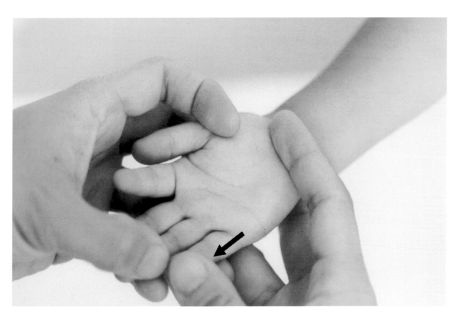

Fig. 7.15

Tui (Liu Fu) 推（六腑） **Pushing (the Six Bowels)**

- With the radial edge of the thumb or the index finger
- Across the ulnar side of the forearm from the medial epicondyle to the wrist
- Approximately 100–300 times
→ **Fig. 7.16**

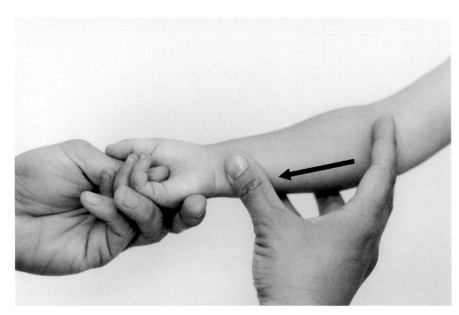

Fig. 7.16

Nausea and Vomiting

Symptoms of Vacuity

Repeated vomiting during eating, sour and foul smell of the vomit, pale facial complexion, cold sensation in the extremities, relief with the application of warmth to the abdomen, soft stools or diarrhea, distention, restless sleep, subdued quiet mood.

Symptoms of Repletion

Immediate vomiting when eating, sour and stinking smell of the vomit, the body feels warm, desire for drinks, restless mood, sharp-smelling stools, intensely-colored urine, distended and painful abdomen.

For Symptoms of Vacuity

Tui (Pi Jing) 推（脾经） **Pushing (the Spleen Channel)**

- With the radial edge of the thumb
- On the radial side of the thumb ascending to the thenar eminence
- Approximately 100–200 times
- → **Fig. 7.17**

Tui (San Guan) 推（三关） **Pushing (the Three Bars)**

- With the thumb
- Ascending from the flexing crease of the hand across the radial side of the forearm up to the elbow
- Approximately 100–200 times
- → See **Fig. 7.7**

Fig. 7.17

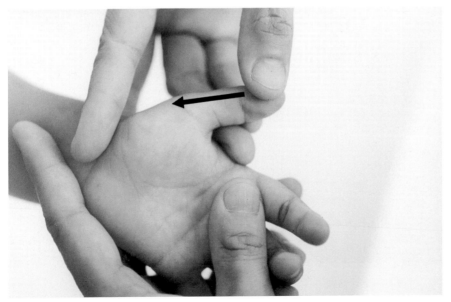

Rou (Tian Shu)   揉（天枢）   **Kneading**
                                (the Celestial Pivot)

- In supine position
- On ST-25 on both sides
- Small circular movements simultaneously with the tips of the index and middle fingers
- Approximately 100–200 times
→ **Fig. 7.18**

Rou (Wai Lao)   揉（外劳）   **Kneading (the Outer**
                                Palace of Toil)

- With the thumb
- On the center of the back of the hand
- Approximately 100–300 times

For Symptoms of Repletion

Xuan Tui (Qing Pi Jing)   旋推   **Rotating Pushing**
                                         (Cleaning the
                           （清脾经）   **Spleen Channel)**

- With the thumb
- On the radial side of the thumb from the thenar eminence to the tip
- Approximately 100–300 times
→ See **Fig. 7.6**

Tui (Liu Fu)   推（六腑）   **Pushing (the Six Bowels)**

- With the thumb
- On the ulnar side of the forearm from the medial epicondyle to the wrist
- Approximately 100–300 times
→ See **Fig. 7.16**

Tui (Qi Jie Gu)   推（七节骨）   **Pushing (the Seventh**
                                   Vertebra)

- In prone position
- With the thumb or index finger
- On the row of spinous processes descending from L4 to the sacrum
- Approximately 100–300 times
→ **Fig. 7.19**

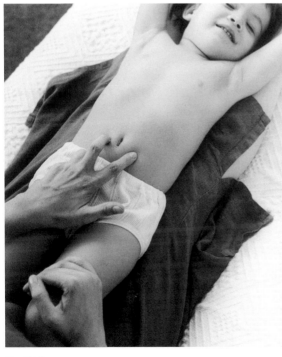

Fig. 7.18

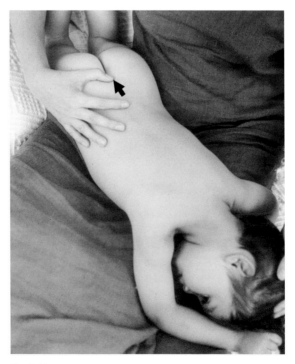

Fig. 7.19

Tui (Tian Zhu Gu)   推（天柱骨）   **Pushing (the Celestial Pivot Bone)**

- In seated position
- With index and middle finger
- On the nuchal line distally. The other hand fixates on the trunk or on the top of the head.
- Approximately 100–500 times
→ **Fig. 7.20**

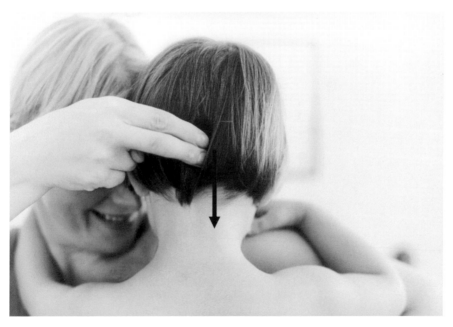

Fig. 7.20

Fever

Symptoms of Vacuity

Headache, sensitivity to cold, congested nose, afternoon fever, warm hands and feet, slender physique and night sweating, lack of appetite.

Symptoms of Repletion

Red face, shortness of breath, lack of appetite, solid stools, restlessness, thirst, desire for drinks.

For Symptoms of Vacuity

Tui (Bu Fei Jing)   推（补肺经）   **Pushing (Supplementing the Lung Channel)**

- With the thumb
- On the gripping surface of the distal phalanx of the ring finger from distal to proximal
- Approximately 100–500 times
- → **Fig. 7.21**

Tui (Tian He Shui)   推（天和水）   **Pushing (Water from Heaven's River)**

- With index and middle finger
- On the volar surface of the forearm from distal to proximal to the elbow
- Approximately 100–500 times
- → See **Fig. 7.1b**

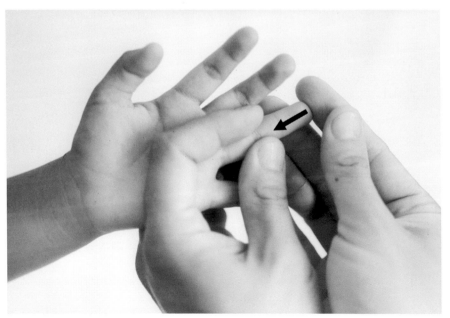

Fig. 7.21

Tui (Tian Men)   推（天门） **Pushing (the Door of Heaven)**

- Alternating with the radial edges of the thumbs, on the GV-channel in the midline from the frontal hairline cranially
- The remaining four fingers are hereby supported on the top of the head.
- Thirty to 50 times

→ **Fig. 7.22**

Rou (Yong Quan)   柔（涌泉） **Kneading (Gushing Spring)**

- With the thumb
- On the proximal edge of the ball of the forefoot on top of the third metatarsal bone
- Fifty to 100 times
- KI-1

→ **Fig. 7.23**

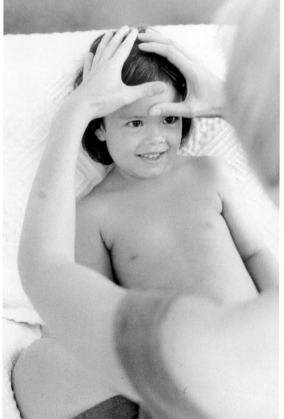

Fig. 7.22

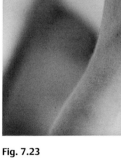

Fig. 7.23

For Symptoms of Repletion

Tui (Qing Fei Jing)   推（清肺经） **Pushing (Clearing the Lung Channel)**

- With the thumb
- On the distal phalanx of the ring finger from proximal to distal
- Approximately 100–500 times
→ See **Fig. 7.21**

Tui (Liu Fu)   推（六腑） **Pushing (the Six Bowels)**

- With the thumb or index finger
- On the ulnar edge of the forearm from proximal to distal
- Approximately 100–500 times
→ See **Fig. 7.16**

Tui (Tian He Shui)   推（天和水） **Pushing (Water from Heaven's River)**

- With the thumb or two fingers
- On the volar surface of the forearm from distal to proximal to the wrist
- Approximately 100 times
→ See **Fig. 7.8**

Bronchitis, Cough, Bronchial Asthma

Tui (Pi Jing)   推（脾经） **Pushing (the Spleen Channel)**

- With the radial edge of the thumb
- On the gripping surface of the distal phalanx of the thumb proximally
- Fifty to 100 times
→ **Fig. 7.24**

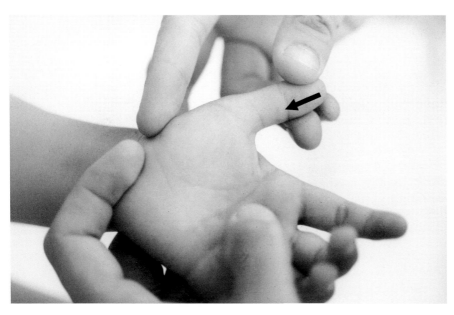

Fig. 7.24

Tui (Qing Fei Jing)　推（清肺经）　**Pushing (Clearing the Lung Channel)**

- With the radial edge of the thumb
- On the gripping surface of the distal phalanx of the ring finger distally
- Fifty to 100 times

Combination of

Rou　揉　**Kneading**

- With thumb or middle finger
- On the point *tan zhong*, which corresponds to CV-17 in adults
- → **Fig. 7.25**

and

Fen Tui　分推　**Lateral Pushing**

- With the thumbs
- In movements emanating from this point, several centimeters to both sides
- Three minutes

Rou　揉　**Kneading**

- In prone position
- With the thumbs
- On the lung point of the bladder channel on both sides of the upper thoracic spine between the upper edges of the shoulder blades
- Fifty to 100 times
- → **Fig. 7.26**

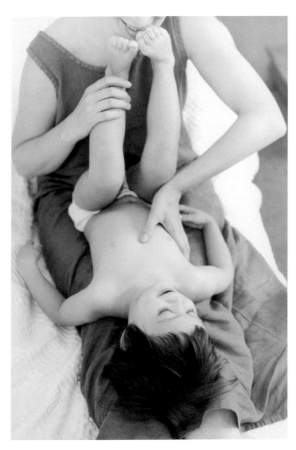

Fig. 7.25

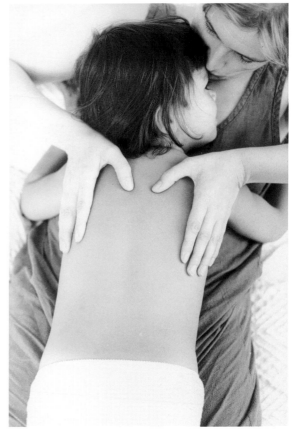

Fig. 7.26

Rou (Tian Tu) 揉（天突） **Kneading (the Celestial Chimney)**

- With the thumbs
- On CV-22 on the upper edge of the sternum
- Three minutes
- → **Fig. 7.27**

Tui (Cuo Mo Xie Lei) 推 （搓摩两肋） **Pushing (Rubbing Both Rib-Sides)**

- With the balls of the hands
- On the seated patient
- Simultaneously across the lateral parts of the belly to the front in the direction of the navel
- Fifty to 100 times
- → **Fig. 7.28**

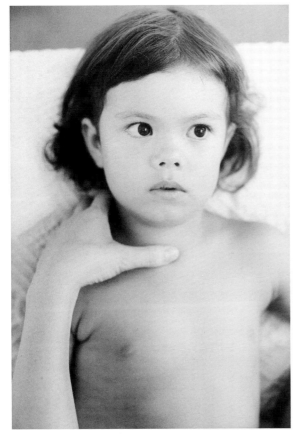

Fig. 7.27

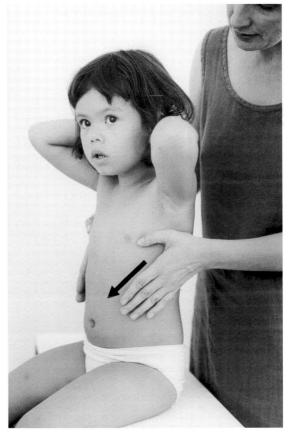

Fig. 7.28

Sleeping Disorders

Symptoms of Vacuity

Lying on the stomach, crying at night, cool extremities, reduced appetite, soft stools, pale face.

Symptoms of Repletion

Lying on the back, crying when the light is turned on, restlessness, intensely colored urine, solid stools, red face and red lips.

For Symptoms of Vacuity

Tui (Pi Jing)　推（脾经）　**Pushing (the Spleen Channel)**

- With the thumb
- On the radial edge of the thumb proximally
- Approximately 100–200 times
→ See **Fig. 7.17**

Tui (San Guan)　推（三关）　**Pushing (the Three Bars)**

- With the edge of the thumb
- Across the radial edge of the forearm to the epicondyle
- Approximately 100–200 times
→ See **Fig. 7.7**

Mo Fu　摩腹　**Round-rubbing the Abdomen**

- With three or four fingers or the entire palm
- Slowly in clockwise direction
- One to 3 minutes
→ See **Fig. 7.10**

For Symptoms of Repletion

Tui (Qing Xin Jing)　推（清心经）　**Pushing (Clearing the Heart Channel)**

- With the thumb
- On the distal phalanx of the middle finger distally
→ **Fig. 7.29**

Then continuing

Tui (Qing Xiao Chang)　推（清小肠）　**Pushing (Clearing the Small Intestine)**

- On the ulnar edge of the little finger distally

and

Tui (Qing Gan Jing)　推（清肝经）　**Pushing (Clearing the Liver Channel)**

- On the distal phalanx of the index finger distally
- Fifty times each

Fig. 7.29

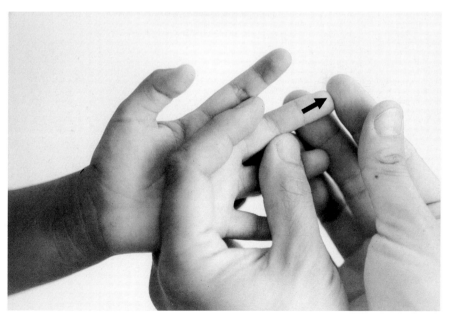

Tui (Qi Jie Gu) 推（七节骨） **Pushing (the Seventh Vertebra)**

- In prone position
- With the thumb
- Descending from L4 in the midline to the sacrum
- Three to five times
→ **Fig. 7.30**

General Stimulating and Strengthening Measures

Tui (Pi Jing) 推（脾经） **Pushing (the Spleen Channel)**

- With the thumb
- On the radial side of the thumb proximally
- Approximately 200–500 times
→ See **Fig. 7.17**

Mo Fu 摩腹 **Round-rubbing the Abdomen**

- With the palm of the hand
- In clockwise direction
- Two to 5 minutes
→ See **Fig. 7.10**

Rou 揉 **Kneading**

- With the thumb
- ST-36 on the ventral proximal lower leg
- Fifty to 100 times
→ **Fig. 7.31**

Na (Nie Ji) 拿（捏脊） **Grasping (Pinching the Spine)**

- With two or three fingers
- In prone position
- On the skin of the back from the sacrum ascending to the neck
- Three to five passes
→ See **Fig. 7.12**

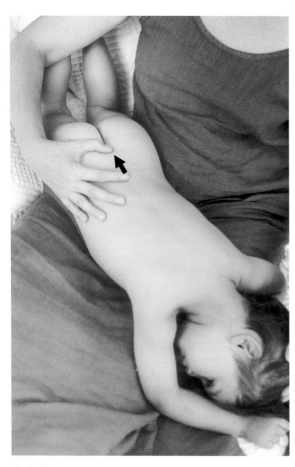

Fig. 7.30

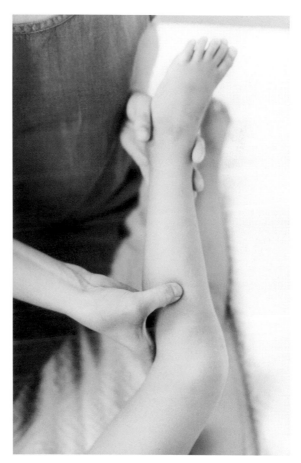

Fig. 7.31

8 Appendix

The Proportional Measurement Based on Finger *Cun*

The basic unit of body-specific measurement—*cun*—to determine distances to other points on the channels and to easily localizable landmarks can be determined as follows:

Thumb measurement: the width of the patient's thumb at the height of the distal joint of the thumb is 1 *cun*.

Middle finger measurement: the tips of the thumb and middle finger are positioned in such a way that they form an O. The distance between the flexing folds of the distal and middle joint of the middle finger is 1 *cun*.

Crossfinger measurements: the width of the index and middle finger at the height of the middle joints is 1.5 *cun*. The width of fingers 2–4 at the height of the middle joint of the index finger is 2 *cun*.

The Selection of Acupressure Points

■ Lung Channel (Fig. 8.1)

LU-1:   1 *cun* below the lateral clavicle, 6 *cun* lateral to
        the midline
LU-2:   immediately medial to the coracoid process
        below the lateral clavicle

LU-7:   proximal to the radial styloid process between
        the tendon of the extensor pollicis and the
        edge of the radius

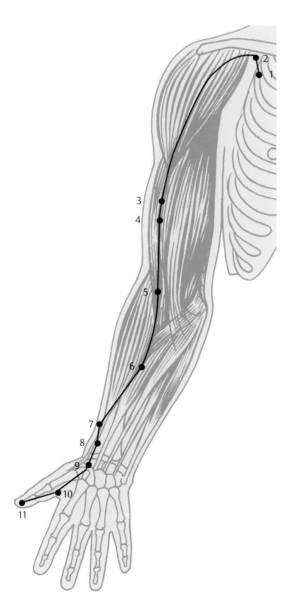

Fig. 8.1

■ Large Intestine Channel (Fig. 8.2)

LI-4:   in the middle of the bisecting line of the angle between metacarpal bones I and II with the thumb abducted

LI-11: in the lateral flexion fold of the elbow joint flexed at 90°, ventral to the lateral epicondyle of the humerus

LI-14: near the humeral insertion of the deltoid, 7 *cun* proximal to LI-11

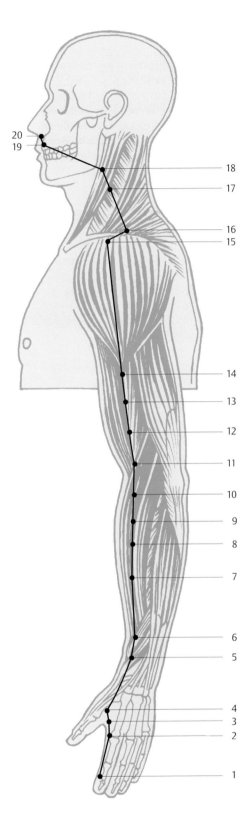

Fig. 8.2

■ Stomach Channel (Fig. 8.3a–c)

ST-2:   on the edge of the zygomatic bone, 1 *cun* vertically below the pupil when staring straight ahead

ST-3:   at the height of the lower border of the wing of the nose, 0.7 *cun* lateral to the nostril

ST-18: vertically below the nipple in the fifth intercostal space, on the medioclavicular line

ST-25: 2 *cun* lateral to the navel

ST-34: 2 *cun* proximal to the lateral upper edge of the patella

ST-36: 3 *cun* below the apex of the patella, 1 *cun* lateral to the edge of the tibia at the height of the tibial tuberosity

ST-37: 3 *cun* distal to ST-36, 1 *cun* lateral to the edge of the tibia

ST-40: in the middle between the apex of the patella and the lateral main arch of the external malleolus, lateroventral above the fibula

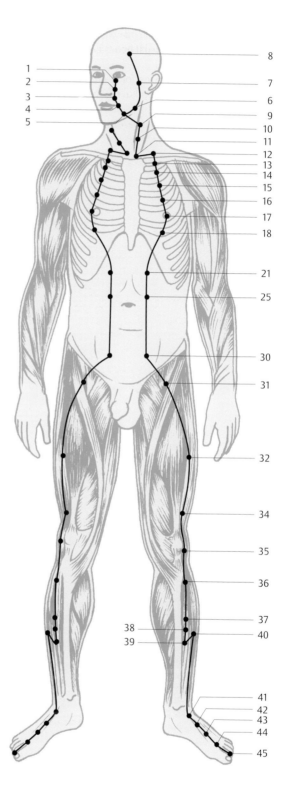

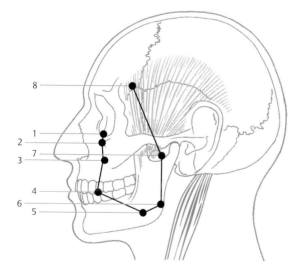

Fig. 8.3a

Fig. 8.3b

ST-41:   on the back of the foot in the middle of the
flexion fold between the tendons of the
extensor hallucis longus and the extensor
digitorum longus

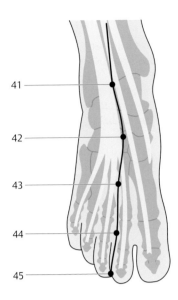

Fig. 8.3c

■ Spleen–Pancreas Channel (Fig. 8.4a, b)

SP-6:   3 *cun* vertically proximal above the internal
         malleolus on the dorsal edge of the tibia

SP-9:   in a depression at the lower edge of the medial
         condyle of the tibia with the knee flexed at 90°

SP-10:   2 *cun* proximal to the upper edge of the patella
         above the medial edge of the patella

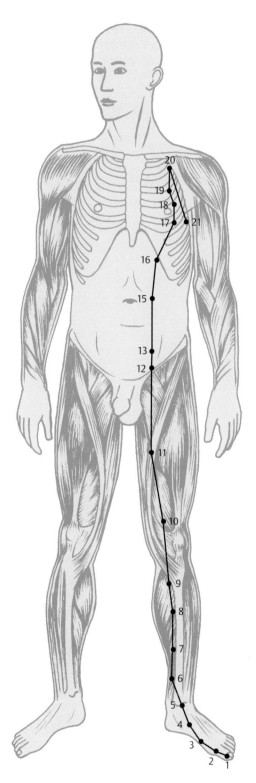

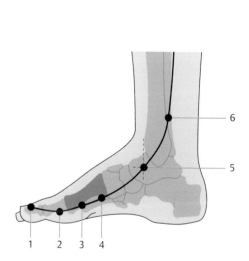

Fig. 8.4a

Fig. 8.4b

■ Heart Channel (Fig. 8.5)

HT-3:   with the elbow flexed at 90°, on the medial end
of the flexion fold of the elbow joint, above the
medial epicondyle of the humerus

HT-7:   proximal and radial to the pisiform bone in the
flexion fold of the hand, radial to the tendon of
the flexor carpi ulnaris

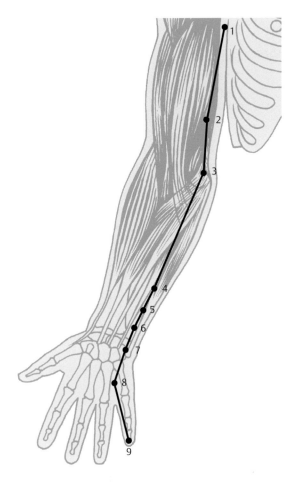

Fig. 8.5

■ Small Intestine Channel (Fig. 8.6)

SI-1:   on the ulnar side of the little finger 0.1 *cun* proximal to the nail angle

SI-3:   proximal to the metacarpophalangeal joint of the little finger by the ulnar tail of the distally located flexion fold of the palm

SI-8:   dorsal to the elbow, in a depression between the ulnar olecranon and the tip of the medial epicondyle of the humerus

SI-10: on the lower edge of the spine of the scapula, vertically above the fold of the armpit

SI-11: in the middle of the infraspinatous fossa of the scapula

SI-14: 3 *cun* lateral to the spinous process of T1, on the levator scapulae near the superior angle

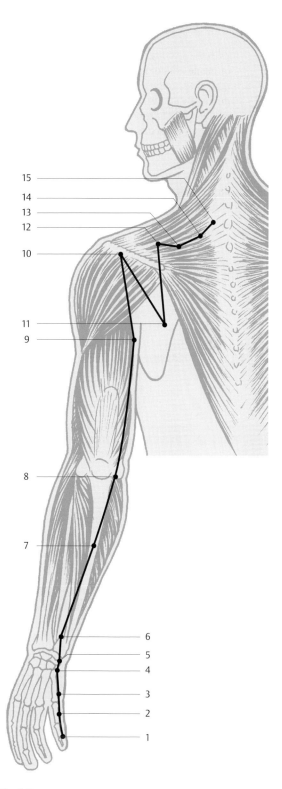

Fig. 8.6

■ Bladder Channel (Fig. 8.7a–d)

BL-1:   in a depression slightly medial and above the medial corner of the eye

BL-2:   on the medial end of the eyebrow, directly above BL-1

BL-4:   1.5 *cun* lateral to the midline of the head, 0.5 *cun* above the hairline at the height of GV-24

BL-7:   1.5 *cun* lateral to the GV channel, 1 *cun* ventral to GV-20, approximately 4 *cun* above the frontal hairline

BL-9:   cranial from the upper edge of the external occipital protuberance, 1.3 *cun* lateral to the GV channel, approximately 2.5 *cun* cranial to BL-10

BL-10:   1.3 *cun* lateral to GV-15, at the height of the interspinous process space C1/2, roughly 0.5 *cun* above the hairline on top of the lateral edge of the trapezius

BL-12:   1.5 *cun* lateral to the spinous process of T2

BL-15:   1.5 *cun* lateral to the spinous process of T5

BL-18:   1.5 *cun* lateral to the spinous process of T9

BL-19:   1.5 *cun* lateral to the spinous process of T10

BL-20:   1.5 *cun* lateral to the spinous process of T11

BL-21:   1.5 *cun* lateral to the spinous process of T12

BL-23:   1.5 *cun* lateral to the spinous process of L2

BL-25:   1.5 *cun* lateral to the spinous process of L4 at the height of the iliac crest

BL-28:   1.5 *cun* lateral to the midline at the height of the second sacral vertebral foramen

BL-29:   1.5 *cun* lateral to the midline at the height of the third sacral vertebral foramen

BL-32:   above the second sacral vertebral foramen

BL-34:   above the fourth sacral vertebral foramen

BL-40:   in the middle of the flexion fold of the knee joint (popliteal fossa) near the popliteal artery

BL-54:   3 *cun* lateral to the midline at the height of the fourth sacral vertebral foramen

BL-57:   in the depression between the gastrocnemius attachments in the middle part of the calves

BL-60:   on the horizontal line in the middle between the lateral malleolus and the Achilles tendon

BL-62:   in a depression by the lower edge of the lateral malleolus

BL-67:   on the fibular side of the little toe, 0.1 *cun* proximal to the nail angle

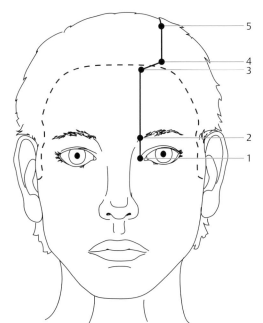

Fig. 8.7a

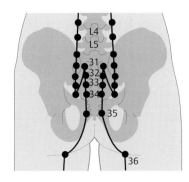

Fig. 8.7b

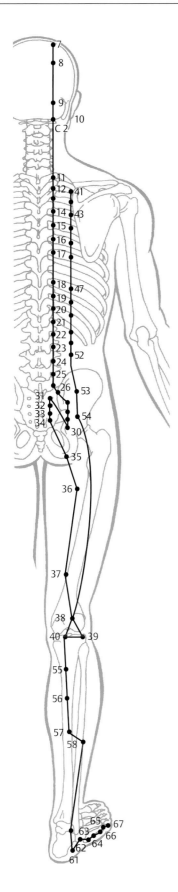

Fig. 8.7c

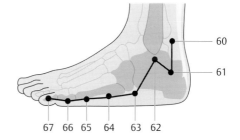

Fig. 8.7d

■   **Kidney Channel (Fig. 8.8a, b)**

KI-1:   in a depression in the sole of the foot between
        the second and third metatarsophalangeal
        joints, roughly on the border between the first
        and second third of the sole (not including the
        toes)
KI-3:   in the middle of a line connecting the medial
        malleolus and the Achilles tendon
KI-6:   directly below the tip of the medial malleolus

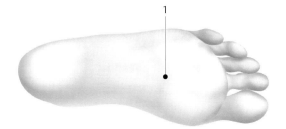

Fig. 8.8a

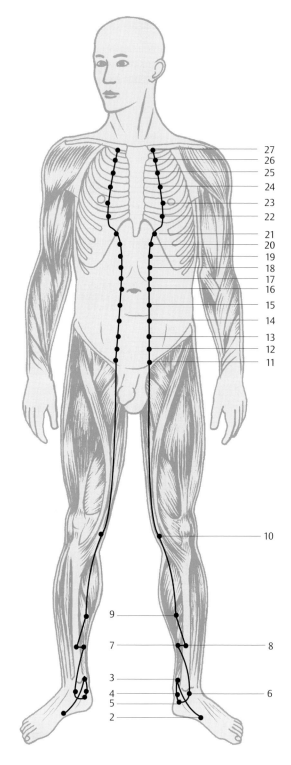

Fig. 8.8b

■ Pericardium Channel (Fig. 8.9)

PC-6:   2 *cun* proximal to the flexion fold of the wrist
         between the tendons of the palmaris longus
         and the flexor carpi radialis

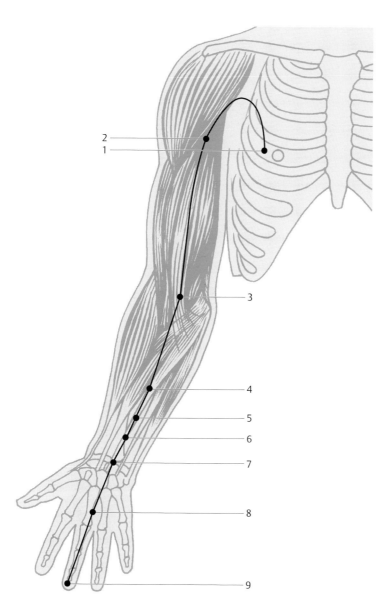

Fig. 8.9

■ Triple Burner (*San Jiao*) Channel (Fig. 8.10a, b)

TB-5:   2 *cun* proximal to the (dorsal) extension fold of the wrist, in the middle of the forearm between radius and ulna

TB-6:   3 *cun* proximal to the (dorsal) extension fold of the wrist, in the middle of the forearm between radius and ulna

TB-14:   in a depression between the acromion and the greater tubercle of the humerus

TB-17:   on the anterior edge of the mastoid process

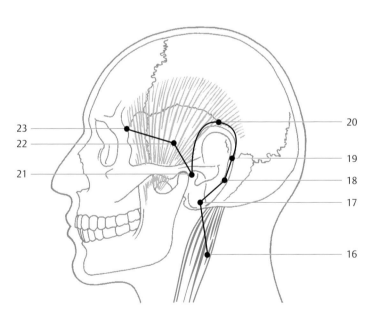

Fig. 8.10a

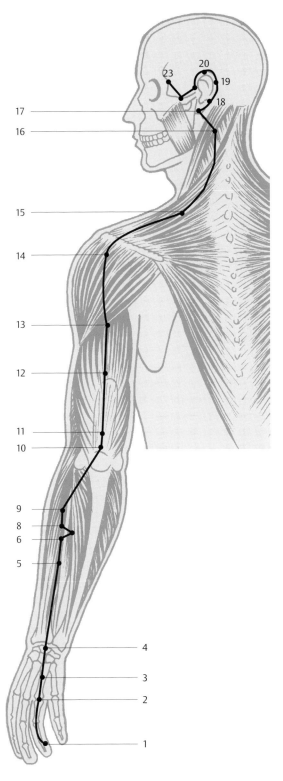

Fig. 8.10b

■ Gallbladder Channel (Fig. 8.11a–c)

GB-12: slightly below and behind the tip of the mastoid process

GB-20: in the depression between the sternocleidomastoideus and trapezius on the occipital bone, at the height of GV-16

GB-21: in the middle of the line connecting the seventh spinous process and the highest point of the acromion

GB-29: on the middle of the line connecting the anterior superior iliac spine and the lateral main arch of the greater trochanter of the femur

GB-30: on the line connecting the greater trochanter to the border of the sacrum and coccyx on the transition from the lateral to the central third of this line

GB-31: on the outside of the thigh, 7 *cun* above the flexion fold of the knee in the standing patient with the arm hanging down, on the place where the tip of the middle finger reaches the iliotibial tract

GB-34: in a depression in front of the head of the fibula

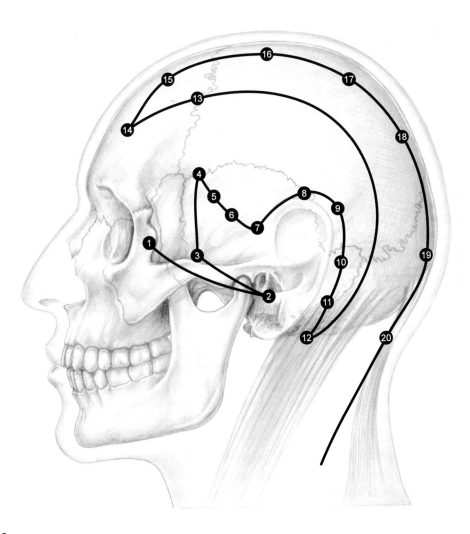

Fig. 8.11a

GB-40: in front of and below the lateral malleolus in a depression lateral to the tendon of the extensor digitorum longus

GB-43: between the fourth and fifth metatarsal bone immediately distal to the metatarsophalangeal joints

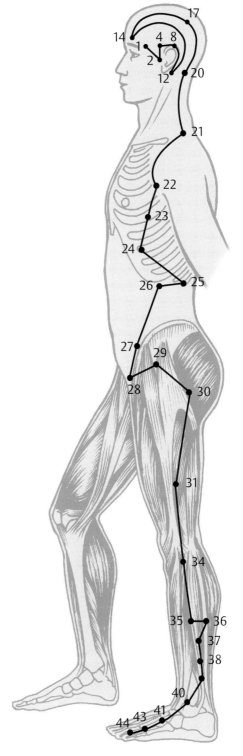

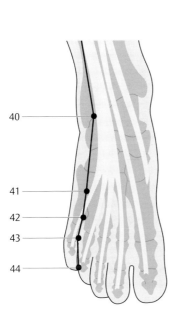

Fig. 8.11b

Fig. 8.11c

■ Liver Channel (Fig. 8.12a, b)

LR-2:   on the proximal end of the webbing between
        the first and second toe

LR-3:   between the first and second metatarsal bone
        in a depression approximately 1.5 *cun* proximal
        to the base joints of the toes

LR-4:   1 *cun* in front of the medial malleolus on the
        tibial side between the tendons of the tibialis
        anterior and the hallucis longus

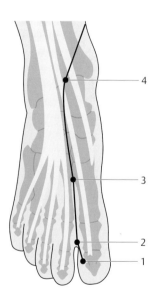

Fig. 8.12a

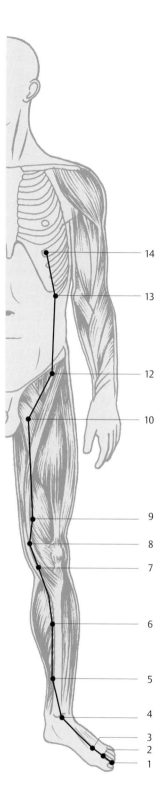

Fig. 8.12b

■ Governing Vessel: *Du Mai* (Fig. 8.13a, b)

GV-4:   below the spinous process of L2

GV-14:   below the spinous process of C7

GV-19:   above the occipital bone, 1.5 *cun* dorsal to GV-20

GV-20:   on the sagittal suture, approximately 7 *cun* from the posterior and 5 *cun* from the anterior hairline, on the line connecting the highest points of the auricles where this line intersects with the midline of the head

GV-23:   1 *cun* cranial to the anterior hairline, 4 *cun* toward the forehead from GV-20

GV-24:   on the midline of the head 0.5 *cun* above the anterior hairline, 4.5 *cun* caudal to GV-20

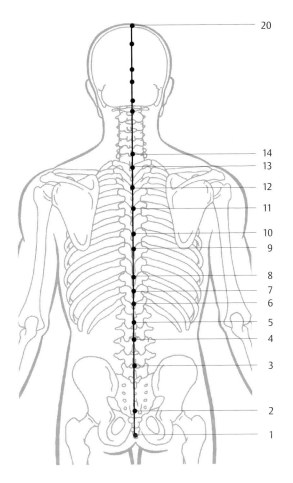

Fig. 8.13a

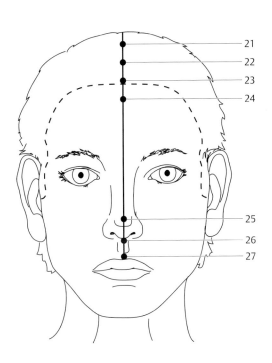

Fig. 8.13b

■ Controlling Vessel: *Ren Mai* (Fig. 8.14)

CV-3:   1 *cun* cranial to the upper edge of the
        symphysis, 4 *cun* caudal to the navel
CV-4:   3 *cun* caudal to the navel
CV-6:   1.5 *cun* caudal to the navel
CV-17: on the sternum at the height of the nipples (i.e.,
        the fourth intercostal space)
CV-22: 1.5 *cun* above the sternum in the middle of the
        suprasternal notch

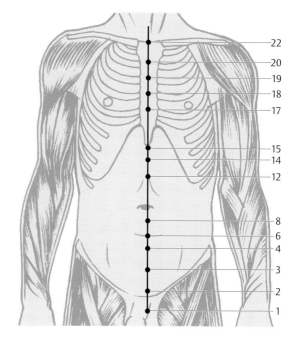

Fig. 8.14

■ Extra Points (Fig. 8.15 a, b)

EX-3: *yin tang*, on the midline between the eyebrows

EX-5: *tai yang*, from the midpoint between the outer corner of the eye and the lateral end of the eyebrow, 1 *cun* to lateral in a depression

EX-54: *an mian*, in the middle between TB-17 and GB-20

Eye points of the back: see the section on the "Spinal Column" in Chapter 2 (p. 31, **Fig. 2.17**)

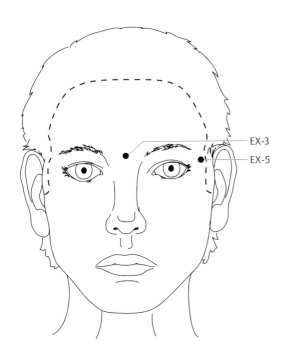

Fig. 8.15a

Fig. 8.15b

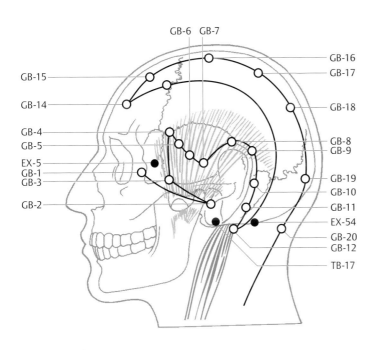

Glossary of *Tuina* Terminology

■ Therapeutic Techniques

Pin Yin	Chinese	English
an	按	pressing (also "acu-pressure")
an ban fa	按扳法	pressing and twisting
an mo	按摩	pressing and rubbing
an xi ti tun fa	按膝提臀法	knee–buttocks counterpressure and circular movement
ban fa	扳法	twisting
ce ban	侧扳	stretching
dou fa	抖法	shaking
dui an	对按	grasping and kneading
fan gong	反功	turning technique
fen tui	分推	lateral pushing
gua	刮	scratching
gun	滚	rolling
heng bo	横拨	transverse frictions
heng ca	横擦	transverse scrubbing
ji	挤	tapping
jing dun	静蹲	isometric strengthening
kua xuan zhuan	旋转法	rotating mobilization of the hip joint
la tui fa	拉推法	pulling and pushing
mo	摩	round-rubbing
mo fu	摩腹	round-rubbing the abdomen
mu jian an	拇尖按	pressing and pushing
na	拿	grasping
na bin	拿髌	patellar mobilization

Pin Yin	Chinese	English
pai	拍	patting
qian	牵	traction
qian la fa	牵拉法	traction and pulling
qian la lü	牵拉将	traction with pushing
qian yin	牵引	traction
qian yin dou fa	牵引抖法	traction with shaking
qian yin lü	牵引将	traction with casting off
qü shen fa	曲伸法	flexion and extension
rou	揉	kneading
shu ca	竖擦	longitudinal scrubbing
si zi	四字	numeral four
ti dou	提抖	traction and shaking
tui	推	pushing
tui an	推按	transverse rubbing
tui liang lei	推两肋	pushing the ribs on both sides
xuan zhuan fa	旋转法	rotating mobilization
xuan zhuan qian yin	旋转牵引	rotating traction
yi shou	意守	concentration and relaxation
zhang ban fa	掌扳	tangential counter-push
zhang dui an	掌对法	pressing

■ Pediatrics

Pin Yin	Chinese	English
fen tui	分推	lateral pushing
mo fu	摩腹	round-rubbing the abdomen
na (nie ji)	拿（捏脊）	grasping (pinching the spine)
rou (dian rou)	揉（点揉）	kneading (point kneading)
rou (tian shu)	揉（天枢）	kneading (the celestial pivot)
rou (tian tu)	揉（天突）	kneading (the celestial chimney)
rou (wai lao)	揉（外劳）	kneading (the outer palace of toil)
rou (yong quan)	柔（涌泉）	kneading (gushing spring)
tui (bu fei jing)	推（补肺经）	pushing (supplementing the lung channel)
tui (cuo mo xie lei)	推（搓摩两肋）	pushing (rubbing both rib-sides)
tui (da chang)	推（大肠）	pushing (the large intestine channel)
tui (liu fu)	推（六腑）	pushing (the six bowels)
tui (pi jing)	推（脾经）	pushing (the spleen channel)
tui (qi jie gu)	推（七节骨）	pushing (the seventh vertebra)
tui (qing da chang)	推（清大肠）	pushing (clearing the large intestine)
tui (qing gan jing)	推（清肝经）	pushing (clearing the liver channel)
tui (qing fei jing)	推（清肺经）	pushing (clearing the lung channel)
tui (qing xiao chang)	推（清小肠）	pushing (clearing the small intestine)

Pin Yin	Chinese	English
tui (qing xin jing)	推（清心经）	pushing (clearing the heart channel)
tui (san guan)	推（三关）	pushing (the three bars)
tui (tian he shui)	推（天和水）	pushing (water from heaven's river)
tui (tian men)	推（天门）	pushing (the door of heaven)
tui (tian zhu gu)	推（天柱骨）	pushing (the celestial pivot bone)
xuan tui	旋推	rotating pushing
xuan tui (bu pi jing)	旋推（补脾经）	rotating pushing (supplementing the spleen channel)
xuan tui (qing pi jing)	旋推（清脾经）	rotating pushing (clearing the spleen channel)

■ Pulse Terminology

Pin Yin	Chinese	English
fu jin	浮紧	floating and tight
hong	洪	surging
hua	滑	slippery
jin	紧	tight
shen	深	deep
shi	实	replete
shuo	数	rapid
xian	弦	stringlike
xi	细	fine
xu	虚	vacuous

Bibliography

Anmo Fachhochschule: China Anmo. 2nd ed. Beijing: Huaxia; 1993

Birch S. Shonishin: Japanese Pediatric Acupuncture. Stuttgart–New York. Thieme Publishers 2011; In press

Chen J. Anatomical Atlas of Chinese Acupuncture Points. 2nd ed. Shandong: Science and Technology Press; 1988

Deng T. Practical Diagnosis in Traditional Chinese Medicine. New York: Churchill Livingstone; 1999

Ergil MC, Ergil KV. Pocket Atlas of Chinese Medicine. Stuttgart–New York: Thieme Publishers; 2009

Fan Y-L. Chinese Pediatric Massage Therapy: A Parent's and Practitioner's Guide to the Treatment and Prevention of Childhood Disease. Boulder: Blue Poppy Press; March 1999

Hempen C-H, Wortman V. Pocket Atlas of Acupuncture. Stuttgart–New York: Thieme Publishers; 2005

Huang J. Naturmedizin—Die medizinische Revolution im 21. Jahrhundert. Taipei: Health Seed; 2000

Ji W. Tuina für Kinder und Säuglinge vor dem Schlafen. Hebei: Wissenschafts- und Technologie Verlag; 1995

Kaptchuk TJ. The Web that has no Weaver: Understanding Chinese Medicine. 2nd ed. New York: McGraw-Hill; 2000

Li J, Wei Y. Chinese Manipulation and Massage: Chinese Manipulative Therapy. Beijing: International Academic Publishers; 1990

Lin ZH. Pocket Atlas of Pulse Diagnosis. Stuttgart–New York: Thieme Publishers; 2007

Luo Y. TCM in der Gynäkologie. Shanghai: Wissenschafts- und Technologie Verlag; 1984

Ma Y, Ma M, Cho Z. Biomedical Acupuncture for Pain Management: An Integrative Approach. New York: Elsevier; 2005

Mehling WE. Atemtherapie [Dissertation Freie Universität Berlin]. Aachen: Shaker; 1999

Padus E. The Complete Guide to Your Emotions and Your Health. Kammaus/USA: Rodale Press; 1992

Porkert M, Zhou J. Premoprehension—Lehrbuch der chinesischen manuellen Therapie. Dinkelscherben: Phainon Edition und Media; 1996

Qü M, Yu C. Practical Sports Medicine. People's Sports. Beijing: Publishing House of China; 2003

Schnorrenberger CC. Chen Chiu: The Original Acupuncture. Boston: Wisdom Publications; 2003

Shanghai TCM-Hochschule: Akupunktur. 3rd ed. Beijing: Volkshygiene; 1986

Sun W. Tui Na. Akupunktur. Theorie und Praxis. 1997;3:239–240

Sun W. Möglichkeiten der TCM bei Tumorpatienten. In: Jehn U (editor). Supportive Therapie. München: Zuckschwerdt; 1998: 45–52

Sun W. Dadi-Qigong. Pocking: Bavaria Bäder-Verlag; 1999

Unschuld P. Huang Di Nei Jing Su Wen: Nature, Knowledge, Imagery in an Ancient Chinese Medical Text. Berkeley, CA: University of California Press; 2003

Wa Z. Zhongguo Yixue Shi (A History of Chinese Medicine). Nanchang: Jiangxi Kexue Jishu;1987

Wa Z. Zhongguo Yixue Shi (A History of Chinese Medicine), Beijing: Renmin Weisheng; 1991

Wang C. TCM in der Kinderheilkunde. Beijing: Volkshygiene; 1998

Wang J. Tuina-Technik-Atlas. 2nd ed. Beijing: Volkshygiene; 1998

Wertsch G, Schrecke BD, Küstner P. Akupunkturatlas. 12th ed. Schorndorf: WBV Biol.-Medizinische Verlagsgesellschaft; 1996

Wühr E. Chinesische Syndromdiagnostik. Kötzting: VGM; 2002

Xia Z. Praktische Akupunktur und Tuina Therapie. Shanghai: Shanghai TCM Hochschule Verlag; 1990

Xie ZF. Classified Dictionary of Traditional Chinese Medicine (New Edition). Beijing: Foreign Language Press; 2002

Yin H. TCM Grundtheorie. Beijing: Volkshygiene; 1989

Yü D. Tuina. 8th ed. Shanghai: Wissenschafts- und Technologie Verlag; 1992

Zhao E: TCM Pulsdiagnose. Tianjing: Wissenschafts- und Technologie Verlag; 1988

Index

Page numbers in *italics* refer to illustrations

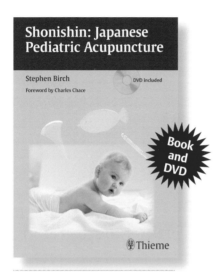
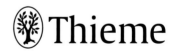

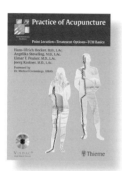
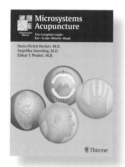
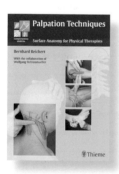
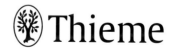

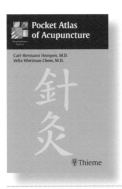
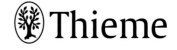